What Every Husband Should Know About Having a Baby

What Every
Husband Shoul
About Havin

Know

a Baby

The Psychoprophylactic Way

Jeannette L. Sasmor, R.N., M.Ed.

Nelson-Hall Chicago

ISBN 911012-18-4

Library of Congress Catalog Card No. 72-75633

For information address
Nelson-Hall Co., Publishers
325 W. Jackson Blvd., Chicago, Ill. 60606

Manufactured in the United States of America

PHOTO CREDITS: page 153, Baby Talk *magazine; page 160, Bob Davidoff; all others, Robert S. De Santo.*

To Jim

who makes life worth sharing

Contents

Foreword

We are living in an era when more and more attention is focused on the problems of social relations between women and men. Understandably, it is still the women who are the more active of the two in presenting and elucidating the issues surrounding the inequalities between women and men.

Where can and should men reveal their concern and desire to help diminish and hopefully eliminate those inequalities? Without minimizing the role men can play politically, socially, and philosophically in establishing equality, we can point to a made-to-order role for the male who wishes to strengthen his family bonds in the face of imminent social change. Certainly those who are interested in achieving a sounder society can do no less than encourage men to join actively in labor and delivery, the processes by which society's basic unit, the family, is expanded.

The relation of man to woman and of woman to man has changed over the centuries: from cave man to our modern civilization; from patriarchal and matriarchal to the present movement toward more equal rights for women—in education, sciences, industry, and, slowly, government. So also are changes manifest in the family. Concomitantly, more women are working outside the home and more men are sharing in the duties of home management.

Because certain relationships have existed for centuries, it does not necessarily follow that they must be fixed forever and that changes cannot or should not occur. Today, more and more efforts are directed toward establishing equal social, political, and economic rights for women. Similar equalities should exist in family relations. When someone is sick, others in the family give of their time and feelings to aid the sick one. Why not the same sharing in a healthy and generally happy situation of childbirth? The child is the product of two people. True, biologically and anatomically the woman bears the child. But it does not follow that a man, after insemination, should do nothing further to assist his wife in childbearing.

In the United States, the concept of family-centered maternity care is spreading. Mutual participation of expectant mother and expectant father is so fully pursued, they are truly acting as a unit. The birth is the concern of that unit with maximum participation of both husband and wife.

From the early nineteenth century, medicine has made rapid progress. Contributions of Lister, Pasteur, Holmes, and Semmelwiess; the growth of understanding of human behavior climaxing in the work of Pavlov and Freud; the advent of anesthesia and analgesia—all raised the life expectancy of mother and child. However, just as in other disciplines, there are blind spots which time and experience uncover. We move forward for a time and then retreat somewhat.

We now know that there are some disadvantages inherent in analgesia and anesthesia. Today more and more obstetricians are decreasing the dosages of analgesia and changing the type and amount of anesthesia because they recognize the potential harm of such modalities for mother and/or child.

A historical sketch will indicate how this retreat came about.

In the 1930s, the great cry among physicians was for increasing supportive measures for women in labor. For many years before and after this, amnesiacs were considered significant supportives. Patients were given such strong analgesics that the resultant amnesia caused other pregnant women to demand such medications. And they were grateful for having been "helped" out of their misery—little knowing about the potential risk of such concentrated doses of medication for mother and child. But when obstetricians begin to limit or even omit medications (saying *sotto voce:* "Better a crying woman than an injured mother or child"), what did they do to replace these medicines? Where was their concern for support of the parturient then?

It took the introduction of Grantly Dick-Read ideas, and then of Pavlovian neuro-physiological concepts, to replace these intensely and widely-used, powerful medical agents. These newly applied psycho-physical methods of prenatal training have been shown to be extraordinary instruments for good since there are no harmful components when they are applied with knowledge and understanding.

In this book, Mrs. Sasmor addresses herself to the role of the husband in the psychoprophylactic method (PPM) of preparation for labor and delivery.

Included in the architecture of the PPM is the use of correctly applied external stimuli—education, deconditioning, exercises, breathing techniques, neuro-muscular relaxation, participation of hospital personnel, and the addition of one of the most powerful agents: the other part of the family unit, the husband.

It is well known that the cerebral cortex influences and determines our conduct, our responses to aural, oral, visual, and physical stimuli. We know the dynamics of the combined stimuli when they act upon an alert cerebral cortex and present a barrier to the strengthening of the conceptualization of the enteroceptive uterine stimuli.

Stated more simply: the patient's greater awareness of her

surroundings and of the cooperation of physicians and other hospital personnel, and her concentrated participation in conscious muscular group relaxation, specific breathing techniques, abdominal massage, and listening to her husband count off the seconds—all are conscious stimuli which interfere with the strengthening awareness of other stimuli coming from the contracting womb.

Important in this dynamic complex of cortical stimuli are the participatory activities of the trained husband during pregnancy, labor, and delivery. His continuing participation with his wife develops in her reflexes conditioned by his presence and activity. It is our profound conviction that such participation by the husband plays a significant role in raising the pain threshold in the parturient. Our experience supports this view. It is one of the positive influences that determine the behavior of the pregnant woman.

Our concept of family-centered maternity care obliges us to include the husband in the method. Since the family is the unit of society, it goes without saying that the husband must take his place in the development, growth, strengthening, and maintenance of the family unit. Our experience in the United States has revealed how true this is.

I know I am treading upon a sensitive area of human relations: the attitude of men towards women. This does not deter me from doing so and elaborating upon it. Men are still the controlling force in human destinies. Throughout most of the world, women are treated as second class citizens. And this applies to maternity care as well. Dr. Fernand Lamaze did a heroic work in bringing PPM to Western Europe. From there it has spread over most of the world. One of his main contributions was his introduction of the husband as an active participant in the preparation of his wife for the birth of their child.

The role of the husband at the side of his wife was rejected by most husbands and—significantly—by most obstetricians. In fact it was even given only lukewarm support by obstetricians pursuing the PPM. Also not enough teachers of the PPM have scheduled the time of their classes to coincide with post work-day hours for those husbands who did wish to participate. I have seen this in my travels in many parts of the world and have been disturbed by it.

It is essentially men who have been responsible for keeping women in subsidiary positions. Obstetricians, being mostly men, have not been exceptions. It seems therefore that those of us who accept the principles inherent in this foreword and in Mrs. Sasmor's book should lead in efforts to erase the social inequalities between men and women, particularly in the area of obstetrical care. And where but in the activities and development of the family unit do we have a more natural opportunity to move in that direction?

When Dr. Lamaze brought PPM to us from the U.S.S.R., he said that man, the husband, *must* be included in the program to give it enduring strength. And most of us in the States who fully accepted the principles laid down by Dr. Lamaze have applied them in our pursuit of the PPM since the organization of the American Society for Psychoprophylaxis in Obstetrics (ASPO) ten years ago.

Why do I feel so impelled to talk and write about the role of the husband in PPM? I was disturbed by what I saw in my travels —in Mexico, Japan, England, and Italy—as well as by what I read in reports from Latin America. Generally, the husband has taken a lesser part in the program. Much of this diminished role is supported by male-chauvinistic rationalization, rationalization often determined by the cultural, economic, and political forces influencing woman's place in society.

Why are husbands playing a more active role in the PPM in the United States? The reasons are 1) historical conditions, 2) shortage of medical and paramedical personnel, and 3) the determination of the ASPO to further the principles of the PPM.

1) *Historical conditions:* It is said that in the United States, the attitude of husbands toward their wives is one of mutual respect and admiration and that there are strong tendencies to achieve equality—all characteristics which tend to cement family units. This is not so in other countries where men hold themselves to be superior to women. Could it not be said that men in those countries speak derisively about American men in *self-defense*—and thus continue in the rut of their own past?

If one accepts this concept of Anthropus Americanus, the foundation already exists for building the home of PPM in the States. Given the stimulus of an alert body of progressive obstetricians to educate expectant mothers in the values of this method, the PPM may look forward to rapid growth here.

2) *Shortage of medical and paramedical personnel:* Increase in the number of trained personnel has not kept pace with population or with the needs of scientific advance. This is especially true in the medical sciences. Cries of distress are heard all over at the inability of hospitals to meet the advances of science because of the shortage of professional and ancillary personnel. More and more women, leaving the warmth of the home and admitted into the hospital, enter a strange wilderness of aloneness and sprouting fears. How horrible to be alone at a critical time in one's life. What atmosphere is more condusive to wild fantasies and illusions of tragic sequence?

On the other hand, how can one measure the emotional, the psychic benefits of the continuous presence of another human being? And how much more value accrues when such a physical presence is that of one's husband? And how also can one measure the gratitude and feelings of relief gained by the overworked medical and paramedical personnel who know that someone, a trained person, is continuously with the parturient, someone who can give an educated response to questions; someone who can report accurately on the character of the labor; someone who can quickly draw medical attention to the needs of the parturient, as well as to the emergence of a possibly dangerous situation? Who but a husband can meet such requirements?

There are those who will counter that a mid-wife or other trained person can serve likewise. They can *if they are available*. But I must add, they can *almost* serve likewise. It is this *almost* that produces a qualitative difference. This *almost* is removed by the presence and participation of a specially trained person—the husband. He is a special person because of his training for a specific event in the lives of two people, himself and his wife. He is a tower of strength for the parturient. He contributes a qualitative component to the patient's activities in labor and delivery of their child; emotionally and supportively toward an easier labor and a healthier child.

Just to see the faces of husband and wife as the child is born is to know that they have gone through a peak experience together, one of mutual rapture, an event never experienced by the deeply drugged parturient or the husband in the waiting room. Only a poet or a musician can describe this esctasy. Such a response is rare in the life of a man or woman and even more rare when it occurs simultaneously in husband and wife.

Psychologists who know the work of Maslow at Brandeis University are familiar with the term "peak experience." From questionnaires, as well as from direct conversations with such couples in the delivery room, we know that few experiences in their lives have so strengthened their love for each other. No other experience has so profoundly increased the respect, admiration, and love of the husband for his wife and of the wife for her husband.

This family-centered maternity care, this mutual participation, spreads its advantages to the child; the physical and emotional needs of the child are satisfied to a greater and more profound degree as the child grows older. And so the benefits go full circle to mother, father, and child. There is statistical evidence supporting this view, as well as the fact that a peak experience rarely occurs in patients who have classical obstetrical management.

3) *Determination of the American Society for Psychoprophylaxis in Obstetrics:* The third condition encouraging the more active participation of the husband in the PPM was the firm determination of the ASPO at its very inception to maintain its basic principles, even as forms of application are modified to meet specific conditions. Fully aware of the causes of deterioration in the Read method *(Childbirth Without Fear)*—largely because even its limited concepts of psycho-physical training were not carried out, we in ASPO pledged ourselves to do everything possible to hold fast to our principles. We do our utmost to prevent the PPM from being diluted by too many compromises.

As one who for years had observed the Read method and noted the increasing variations and as the first president of ASPO, I have led a continuing fight to prevent adulteration of the PPM. This has been evident in our literature, in our guidelines for teachers and public meetings, and in the practices of associated obstetricians.

Our most difficult problem has been in obtaining permission for the husband to be present in the delivery room. It is, nevertheless, important to know that, with one exception, wherever we did get permission, it has never been rescinded. The one exception was a hospital in which the directorship changed and family-centered care was not a part of the new director's philosophy.

At the first national convention of ASPO in 1967, Dr. Luis Bernal A. Castroverde of Puerto Rico spoke about the father's part in pregnancy and childbirth in the PPM. He pointed out the usual cliches about a man in this situation, for example: "This is woman's business." Obstetricians fostered this view and did nothing to probe these absurd ideas, making matters worse by their indifference. The husband took his wife to the hospital "worried and ignorant, with only one thing on his mind 'how great will be her suffering, poor thing.' His attempts at reassurance were hollow and without conviction because he did not really know what to say."

Dr. Castroverde drew attention to the school of reflexology which gave its scientific label to the method: the PPM. He kept written testimonies of variously expressed opinions of happy fathers, written and tape-recorded. He pointed out that a well-prepared husband is a useful and capable person. One comment by a husband is significant: "I was feeling more like a father, as if I were more of a man."

Dr. Castroverde continued: "Such a husband transmits to his wife a feeling of security and confidence because of his presence and positive attitude . . . . The husband becomes the affective and effective liaison between his wife, the obstetrician, and the preparation team. Throughout the training he acts like a coach, a teacher's assistant, and even the obstetrician's aid during delivery—particularly because of his coaching and his ability to report accurately to the doctor. His is not a passive presence. To his wife, he is really her husband and the father of her child."

Finally, I shall briefly report a study supporting our view that there are psychological advantages for both husband and wife because of husband participation in the PPM. This study, "The Psychology of Pregnancy and Childbirth: An Investigation of Natural Childbirth," by Dr. Deborah Tanzer, was a five year prospective effort comparing a group of PPM-trained women with a control group following classical methods of care.

Great differences were noted in the descriptions by the two groups—in tone and content. For the PPM group there were descriptions of joint participation in activity; togetherness in the delivery room during and after birth; excitement by husband and wife and the development of "peak experience" for both of them. In the wife, there were changes of perception of her relationship with her husband. The control group largely limited themselves to statements that were mostly negative in tone.

On the broader question in psychology of the husband's

presence at delivery, thoughts of male-female differences or differences in masculinity and femininity were less frequent than thoughts regarding childbirth. The concept of a male identification with childbirth came from many sources such as psychoanalytic formulations, facts about couvade, facts about the high incidence of psychogenic, pregnancy-stimulated symptoms and other illnesses among men during their wives' pregnancy. We however saw that male involvement with childbirth need not result in de-masculinization as so often has been described.

Indeed, the opposite was true: actually the PPM-trained husbands were strong, competent, in charge, capable of being leaned upon, and dependable, and they possessed other traditional aspects of masculinity *without detracting from or limiting the role of the wife*. The husband was involved, working hard, and surprised at his own feelings of nonsqueamishness. For the control group, husbands were seen as incompetent. They got in the way or needed "taking care of." And this produced feelings of superiority or condescension in their wives.

I conclude by quoting part of a letter from a happy father.

"We owe a lot to psychoprophylaxis. Perhaps this report can repay in part. Perhaps it can encourage other couples to try this method. There is more to gain than just the conquest of fears and controlled delivery. There is an intense emotion beyond anything else people can experience in a lifetime. When you are with your wife at the moment of your child's birth, the *exchange of love is indescribable*. I must admit that when I had agreed to attend classes I felt out of place. I had thought that was a woman's business. And until the last hour of delivery I seemed to be walking in a taboo area. But now I laugh at it all and pity the man who fears it."

BENJAMIN SEGAL, M.D., F.A.C.S.

Consulting Gynecologist-Obstetrician, Lincoln Hospital, New York City;
Former President, The American Society for Psychoprophylaxis in Obstetrics.

Acknowledgments

This book is a result of long-held beliefs that husbands are interested and would like to participate more in many areas of family life, especially in the birth of their children. I would like to thank all those husbands who in the past ten years throughout this country have proved that this is the case by joining with their wives in classes on prepared childbirth and by coaching their wives in labor and delivery.

My sincere thanks also to those forward-looking physicians who have accepted fathers as members of the obstetrical team and recognized their importance as labor coaches.

I would like to thank those qualified childbirth educators, who have worked tirelessly and diligently in the preparation of teachers who recognize the role of the husband and can adequately prepare husbands to assume their roles competently during childbirth. Most especially, I would like to acknowledge here the efforts of Constance R. Castor, R.N., B.S., for having designed and administered an ongoing program of professional preparation for childbirth educators. With her associates, Polly De Santo, R.P.T., and Patricia Hassid, R.N., Mrs. Castor has moved childbirth education beyond technical training to a profession which prepares couples to assume their proper roles on the obstetrical team without fanaticism.

I would like to thank my distinguished colleague Patricia Hassid, R.N., for another service. It has been her intelligent comments and suggestions which have guided me throughout the writing of this book. From her wide experience and that of her husband Dr. Roger Hassid, an obstetrician, many of my ideas have been verified.

Finally and most importantly, I want to thank my husband Jim without whose encouragement and support this book would never have been written.

Introduction

This book is intended for every father-to-be. For generations, the man approaching fatherhood has been completely ignored while attention is heaped upon his pregnant spouse as though pregnancy were her own, unshared accomplishment. This attitude totally underestimates the contributions that the husband can and should make to the bearing of their child. This situation is rapidly changing for the better. Husbands throughout the country are demanding the opportunity to act as partners and to undertake parenthood as their wives do, at the start of and during the long months of pregnancy. They are asking to participate in the labor and delivery processes, sharing the experience of the birth of their children with their wives.

This book is intended for the prospective father. It explores the emotional pitfalls of pregnancy and offers constructive suggestions which may serve to make the experience of having a baby one which will bring the partners into a new relationship of deeper understanding. It also looks at the labor and delivery situation, not as one to be feared and avoided by the father, but as one which the couple can train themselves to meet with control and dignity. And, finally, it looks at the new family and some of the adjustments that will have to be made after the birth of the baby.

The expectant father can make significant contributions to his wife and his marriage during the time he and she are awaiting the arrival of their baby. This book is designed to help him to recognize some of the landmarks of the childbearing cycle and to respond to these developing situations in a way that will be effective in furthering the kind of husband-wife-family relationship one hopes for when he gets married.

1

You and Your Pregnant Wife

So your wife is pregnant! You are going to be a father! How great! (It is awful.) How exciting! (It is depressing.) You are going to be a family. (What have I gotten myself into?)

If you find yourself feeling all of the above, alternately or at the same time, you are among the majority of fathers-to-be. Most intelligent, sensitive men feel the great joy of fatherhood, but at the same time they are almost overwhelmed by a sense of responsibility. This is a normal reaction to the coming change in your family. You as a husband *are* responsible morally and legally for your wife and your children.

One of the ways that nature forces man to mobilize his strengths is to produce just the kind of anxiety you are experiencing. To relieve the anxiety one must make decisions and take action. So it is with the expectant father. Unless it is your intention to sit out this pregnancy as a silent partner, you too will be taking a long look at your life and your hopes and your wife and her dreams. Together you will begin to make long-range plans for your unborn child. And, just as important, you will plan for your wife's pregnancy and the birth of your child together.

Are you surprised that I am suggesting that you, a husband, will assume a role in having this baby? Well, do not be. As a husband and father, you have a right to be a part of this. As you exercise your right, you can make a contribution to your wife, to yourself, to your baby, and to your marriage. It is your right to act as a husband and an expectant father in assisting your wife to plan for the birth of your child.

For generations, having babies and raising children have been considered strictly woman's work. This is not true any more. Husbands all over America are taking an active part in the period of expectation. These husbands are demanding the right to be partners, to act as fathers of the babies and supporters of the families.

There are many opportunities during the pregnancy for you to extend yourself in ways that will make you an important part of having your child and in which you and your wife can share the burdens and joys of childbearing. And many of these opportunities are outgrowths of just being a husband. What you need to know is how you fit into the whole childbearing picture and what exactly you can do.

Husbands have always been as ignorant as their wives about reproduction. For this reason, they sometimes fearfully avoid taking part in the birth of their children. Professionals tend to interpret this fearful avoidance as disinterest. Coupled with the intense mid-Victorian, puritanical determination to segregate the sexes, this attitude has developed a tradition of medical care during pregnancy which isolates husband from wife. Not only is this ridiculous, it is inhumane.

Pregnancy and childbearing are normal, healthy processes. Even though the pregnant woman is brought to a center of medical knowledge to have her pregnancy managed and not to be treated for some disease, she is cared for as any sick person, isolated from her husband and put to bed. This is no longer acceptable to a large portion of our population. Families want to be treated as families. Most husbands are concerned about and interested in their wives' pregnancies, and they can be invaluable during this period of expectancy if they are given enough information about what kind of action is appropriate.

There are many milestones during the nine month wait. Each will be manifested in a change in your wife. Each represents a step forward. Recognizing the milestone is half the game for the husband. And helping your wife to cope at each step along the way is the rest of the ballgame.

Your wife is not going to change drastically just because she is pregnant. And you of all people know her moods best. You will find her traits, the things about her that endear her to you, will be exaggerated just because she *is* pregnant. If your wife tends to be quick-witted and glib, you may find yourself on the receiving end of her sarcasm. If she tends to be vain, she may be overly concerned about the changes in her appearance. If she cries at movies, she may cry at nothing in particular. Nobody can predict how your own wife will behave when she becomes pregnant. But whatever idiosyncrasies develop, be assured that they will disappear after the baby is born.

CHOOSING AN OBSTETRICIAN

The first decision that you and she will need to make together is choosing an obstetrician. If made unwisely or without proper information, it may be the last decision you make together for the duration of the pregnancy. You and your wife must look closely at what you expect to get out of the experience of having a baby. If all you want is a baby, then any competent obstetrician will do.

However, your decision to share childbearing with your wife means that you must find an obstetrician who accepts you, the husband, as part of the team. There are almost as many schools of obstetrical practice as there are of psychiatry. But there are two definite ways for you to find a doctor who practices family-centered obstetrics.

First way: interviewing

The first way is interviewing, which can be a costly adventure. It requires that you and your wife make an appointment with a physician. The three of you sit down and discuss the doctor's point of view. You can ask him how he feels about husbands coming with their wives for office visits. This is often not possible in practice because of most husbands' work schedules. But the doctor's answer can be revealing. You can ask how he feels about prepared childbirth. And, finally, you should ask what he sees as the role of the husband in labor and delivery.

Interviewing in this manner reveals more in attitudes than in information. Some doctors will not see you at all, talking only to your wife. Others will tell you right away that they do not permit husbands in labor or delivery for a variety of reasons. Still others are more subtle, and you need to be keenly observant during interviews with these.

The physician who tells you not to worry, to leave everything to him, is one to whom the thinking couple will want to leave nothing. He is autocratic and will deliver your baby as he has delivered babies for many years without regard for what he considers to be the whims of lay people. The doctor who gives you vague answers, no matter how pleasant, should also be avoided. He does not know what you are really asking, and chances are he is not informed about husband participatory childbirth.

This does not negate the obstetrical competence of these men. It only tells you that for the kind of experience you and your wife are seeking, they are not suitable. The obstetrician for you is the one who is not uncomfortable with your questions and who offers suggestions about how you can best help your wife during pregnancy. He will also practice in a hospital which allows husbands in the labor room at least and hopefully in the delivery room.

The reason that this kind of interviewing is costly is that you are actually making an office visit. The only things the doctor has to sell are time, knowledge, and skills. You are seeking each. Therefore, he is entitled to a fee for an office visit. One should be warned however that the interview must come before an examination. The examination entitles the physician to a fee substantially higher than one for an interview.

Second way: ASPO, ASCE

The second way to find an obstetrician who practices family-centered care is far easier than interviewing and less costly. There are national organizations with member physicians who recognize the importance of the husband to the obstetrical team. By writing these organizations you can obtain the name and location of the physician nearest you. They are: The American Society for Psychoprophylaxis in Obstetrics, Inc., 7 West 96 Street, N.Y., N.Y. 10025, and The American Society of Childbirth Educators, Inc., 230 Riverside Drive, N.Y., N.Y. 10025.

Membership in the physicians divisions of ASPO and ASCE is only open to qualified physicians, the majority of whom meet the requirements for certification by the American Board of Obstetricians and Gynecologists. This tells you that they are competent practitioners. The organizations are dedicated to spreading the psychoprophylactic method of preparation for childbirth, which has become synonymous in this country with husband participatory labor and delivery. You can play an active role with one of these doctors. Unfortunately, ASPO and ASCE physicians are not yet in every area of the United States. In those areas where there is none, you will have to find your doctor through interviewing.

Having found a cooperative physician, you have taken the first step toward a shared childbirth. If you already have an obstetrician as you read this, it is important that you interview him with the same ends in mind. Many times doctors are chosen on the recommendations of friends and relatives who may not have been seeking the same experience.

If you and your wife are earnest about sharing your child's birth, you must talk to your doctor. He may be in favor, or he may not. He is not a mind reader and cannot know your intention unless he is told. And you must know his attitudes in order to make an intelligent decision about whether or not to continue with him.

It is a shame to go along supposing that your kind, understanding obstetrician sees things your way only to be grossly disappointed when your wife arrives in labor. You and your wife *must* talk to him, initially to identify his attitudes and throughout the pregnancy to be sure he understands what you two expect.

FACTS ABOUT REPRODUCTION

Once you have an obstetrician, you and your wife should get down to the business of learning about having a baby. It is amazing in an age so advanced technologically that man in general knows so little about the natural functions of his body. Reproduction is a normal process. Yet, because the subject of S-E-X was taboo for so many generations, modern man is incredibly ignorant and superstitious about childbearing. Some facts about the nature of human reproduction are essential if you are to understand the later stages of pregnancy.

Obvious to one and all are the physical differences between women and men. These differences are more than skin deep. Our bodies function through an intricate system of chemical balances, each organ governed by the secretion of a hormone. In your internal reproductive organs, or testes, a hormone, testosterone, is produced. It is this hormone which gives you the masculine characteristics of a deep voice and a beard.

Your wife's internal reproductive organs, or ovaries, produce hormones, estrogens, which give her a high voice and developed breasts. While you are capable of impregnating your wife at almost any time you have intercourse, she is not always ready to become pregnant. Your testes are continually producing spermatozoa. But your wife only produces one egg, or ovum, a month.

She can only become pregnant at the time during the month when an egg has been released from her ovary and is travelling through the Fallopian tubes which bridge the ovary and the uterus. If the ovum is not fertilized on its way to the uterus, it will pass out of her body. The uterus no longer needs the extra blood supply and tissue it has built up to receive the fertilized egg. They will be discharged during her menstrual period.

Estimating birth date

Because most women have twenty-eight day cycles from the beginning of one menstrual period to the beginning of the next, the date of your baby's birth is estimated by the date of your wife's last menstrual period. Ovulation, or the release of the egg from the ovary, usually occurs some time between the tenth and sixteenth day of the cycle. Fertilization must occur some time before thirty-six hours after ovulation or the unfertilized egg will pass out of the body. This situation allows the semiscientific estimation of delivery by using the formula:

Date of last menstrual period minus three months plus seven days equals estimated date of confinement (LMP – three months + seven days = EDC).

However, not every woman does have a menstrual cycle of exactly twenty-eight days. This formula can be off by as much as two weeks in either direction. Your baby can be born two weeks before or two weeks after the estimated delivery date. Your obstetrician can give you a better estimate as the due date approaches since he can determine the approximate size of the baby.

Once your wife has become pregnant, the chemical balance in her body undergoes a change. Her body begins to secrete a hormone, progesterone, necessary to maintain the pregnancy. Without this hormone as a signal to her body that she is pregnant, your wife's uterus would shed its lining as it did in previous months. But the presence of progesterone causes the "missed period," usually the first indication that you are going to be a parent. It is also the presence of progesterone that leads to the other symptoms and some of the discomforts of pregnancy.

THE FIRST TRIMESTER

The first trimester, or first three months of pregnancy, are really the most difficult for the majority of couples. This is truly the period of adjustment. You will both be examining and re-examining your feelings about your coming child. It is not unusual in these early months for couples to have negative feelings toward the pregnancy. This does not make you bad parents.

After all, the unborn child does represent a threat to your status quo. You know just what a comfortable life you and your wife are sharing. What kinds of changes will this interloper cause? Mothers-to-be often experience a let's-forget-the-whole-thing feeling. Outright rejection of the pregnancy for whatever stated reason, comfort, financial, social, is common among women in the early months. They are experiencing all of the unpleasantness of a changing body without any of the rewards of actually sensing a life within.

Fathers-to-be have been studied much less in these first three months. However, the expectant father is plagued by his own negative feelings. Just as his wife, he is experiencing second thoughts. Not only is he doubting the wisdom of having a child now, but he is looking at how miserable pregnancy has made his wife. You are apt to be feeling very unhappy because as a responsible husband you no doubt will accept full blame for every twinge your wife reports. Well, you are half right.

Always remember, having a baby requires a partnership. You were both there at the beginning! Now she is feeling down with the symptoms of pregnancy. Both of you sitting around feeling sorry for her will accomplish nothing except to make you feel more guilty. There are many things you can do to help your wife through this difficult period. By helping her, you will be helping both of you. If you take an active part in this pregnancy, you will find that you and your wife will understand each other even better than before and have more to offer your baby.

You may be wondering how you can do anything when the pregnancy is *inside* your wife. The answer is obvious. You cannot do a thing about the pregnancy. What you can do is anticipate in what way the pregnancy will be affecting her and then take action to make her more comfortable. With all the emphasis on medical management, we often forget that pregnancy is a normal process which follows a predictable pattern. This is especially easy to forget when it is *your* wife who is pregnant with *your* child.

Emotional reactions

Most couples do share common feelings. However, because they rarely discuss their reactions with friends or relatives, these reactions seem unique to each couple. Nevertheless, pregnancy is predictable. If you are to be most effective, you will need to know the general patterns and major milestones of each trimester.

Pregnancy is described in three trimesters. This is useful to you in gaining an overall picture of pregnancy. Each trimester has its own peculiar pleasures and problems. By learning the general pattern, you will know approximately what to expect and what you can do.

It should be mentioned here that each pregnancy is unique

in detail but alike in pattern. Do not look for every minor detail of pregnancy mentioned in this book to take place in your wife. Even the same woman pregnant for the second time may have an experience different from her first. Get to know the general pattern of pregnancy, and then look at your wife in the light of this knowledge to see where she is without trying to force her to fit into a preconceived notion of what pregnancy ought to be.

As mentioned before, the first trimester is usually the most difficult. The answer to whether those first three months will be remembered with groans or will mark the beginning of a newer and deeper understanding between you two rests almost entirely with you, the husband.

Dealing with guilt

All our lives we are taught not to speak of our feelings. We learn to be inhibited. As a result, when pregnancy occurs and couples feel the normal fears and doubts, they hide these thoughts in the deepest, darkest recesses of their minds to ferment there into full-blown feelings of guilt. Feeling guilty about reacting in a normal human way can mar not only the first trimester but the rest of the pregnancy, causing unnecessary tension for both mother- and father-to-be. You can help to avoid this.

In fact, there is a great deal that you can do to make this pregnancy the best possible one for your wife and yourself by anticipating just such bad developments and attempting to avoid their occurrence. It is true that no act of man is going to allow you to carry or deliver this baby. That is entirely your wife's responsibility. But your responsibility is to guide her and support her in the same way a coach serves a team. For this job there is nobody as well equipped as you. You know your wife better than any other person in the world. And you have a vested interest in this pregnancy. All that you need to be a successful coach are a few guidelines to help you recognize the major milestones of each trimester.

Initiating discussion

The first milestone that you will meet will be the emotional reactions commented upon. To cope most effectively with these reactions, both your wife's and your own, you are going to have to initiate discussion. You are probably thinking that you and she discuss things all the time and that this is a silly suggestion. Remember, all our lives we are taught not to share our secret thoughts. People may laugh at us or say we are crazy or think we are perverted or bad. You may even feel silly when you start to talk about how you feel.

If you and your wife are not really accustomed to talking seriously about your feelings, she may even misinterpret what you are trying to say. This is where the true coach steps in. You will probably have to meet her more than halfway, first by initiating the discussion and then by anticipating her possible misunderstanding. It is up to you to see that she does not get the wrong idea. You are not sorry that she is pregnant. You do not blame her; it is not her fault that she is pregnant.

Admitting this is the first step toward a mutual understanding that many couples celebrating their fiftieth anniversary never achieve. Talking freely is not an easy thing for civilized human beings to do. It requires that you act with courage. You must be willing to try to guide your wife into a revealing conversation. You will have to take the first step. It is a giant step, granted, but one that will help you and your wife to work together for the rest of the pregnancy and through the rest of your marriage.

Anticipating change

The second milestone of these three months is more obvious because it involves a physical change. It is often a period of endurance which lasts, thank goodness, for only the first trimester. While there may be little visual evidence on the outside for some time, there are many changes going on within your wife. This is a time when you will need to look at all your immediate plans with a little deliberate forethought so that you can include all the details that will make this period more pleasant for her.

You will be acting not only for her. Looking at it from a purely selfish point of view, there is no one more miserable than a man whose wife is out of sorts. Therefore, to help you to be more able to anticipate the possible problems of the first trimester, it would be useful to look at the changes that do occur.

To assist her to carry and deliver your child, your wife's body will undergo many changes, internally and externally. Many of the internal changes occur within the first trimester. It will take her almost the full three months to adjust to the changes within.

Morning sickness

Probably the most frequent complaint experienced by almost fifty percent of all pregnant women is morning sickness. It is often the result of the natural phenomena of early pregnancy. The reproductive organs produce larger amounts of hormones, the chemicals which regulate the body systems. These particular hormones are necessary for pregnancy. In addition, the motility (power to move spontaneously) of the stomach tends to decrease as does the amount of free hydrochloric acid in the stomach. This combination often results in nausea, which frequently occurs in the morning. It can occur at any time during the day, but most women experience the most annoying sensations upon arising.

You can help with this problem by making your wife's mornings less hectic. Encourage her to stay in bed when you get up. Keep either plain soda crackers or dry toast at the bedside and have her munch on one when she awakens. After she has her crackers, she should stay in bed for at least half an hour. This may mean some change in your morning schedule to make her staying in bed seem convenient. But, in most cases, if this is done, by the time your wife gets up and can sit down to a cup of coffee with you, she will be able to enjoy it and keep it down.

A word of caution: it is especially helpful for you to make an effort to prevent your wife from developing a pattern of nausea and vomiting. For while morning sickness is physiologically caused, its pattern is very difficult to eliminate once it has begun. Your wife can become extremely uncomfortable if this pattern is established. She may be unable to keep any food on her stomach for the greater part of the first trimester.

Outward changes

Even in the early part of her pregnancy, you may notice some small changes in your wife's body. Most men see their wives as becoming more womanly in shape. Because her body is preparing itself not only for carrying and giving birth but also for nurturing the baby after birth, you will probably see a decided increase in the size of your wife's breasts. Many husbands are more than a little pleased by this development. However, enlarging breasts can be quite sensitive to the touch. If you tend to be a squeezer, this is the time for you to find some other way to express your affection.

Your wife may not share your enthusiasm about this change either. Should she be less than pleased by your compliments to her blossoming figure, you would do well to remain a silent admirer. The changes will remain at least for the duration of the pregnancy and should she breastfeed, for that length thereafter.

Another change of the first trimester is the direct physical result of the enlarging uterus not yet moving upward in the abdominal cavity. Consequently, when it expands in all directions it leaves less room for the other body organs in the pelvic area. This means that the bladder which normally can expand to hold a half day's supply of urine has less room for expansion. For this reason your wife is constantly in search of a ladies room. You can help her most with this inconvenience by planning ahead.

Obviously this is no problem at home. But the wise husband will choose restaurants and theaters that have easily accessible facilities. Likewise, when you are thinking of a drive, even one you would normally make without stops, you would do well to plan your route so that rest stations are never more than a few minutes away. Your wife will appreciate your thoughtfulness.

THE SECOND TRIMESTER

What we have been discussing are the early signs of pregnancy. As your wife moves on to the next trimester, you and she will experience a whole new set of reactions. Around the beginning of the fourth month, your wife will begin to feel human again. You will be relieved to see her normal good spirits returning. Many of the complaints of the first three months will temporarily disappear. You and she will probably spend most of the fourth month just enjoying each other's company. Without the discomforts of pregnancy plaguing you, you can again focus on the happy plans for the baby. Also, you can help your wife get back on her regular schedule which probably went by the board in those first three months.

Quickening

Toward the end of the fourth or beginning of the fifth month, your wife may experience a fluttering sensation deep within her lower abdomen. This is the growing fetus moving. Although the fetus moves throughout pregnancy, your wife will not be aware of the sensation, known as quickening, until the fetus is large enough to make himself known. Even as quickening takes place, the sensation is not yet strong enough for you to feel from the outside. Nevertheless, you and she will still share the excitement of knowing that your baby is alive and well and growing inside your wife.

About the same time, the doctor will be able to hear the baby's heartbeat without any elaborate electronic equipment. This is the time that you and your wife begin to really feel that you *are* going to have a baby. Until this point, all seems just a series of inconvenient unpleasantries for your wife. But from this time onward, pregnancy means that there is a real, live baby about to enter your lives.

The kinds of complaints expressed in the second trimester are usually minor compared with the awe and excitement most couples experience. The physical discomforts are a result of the decreased motility of the gastro-intestinal tract and the pressure caused by the growing uterus as it rises upward into the abdominal cavity. One complaint is constipation. Others are heartburn and flatulence. The preferable way to deal with these problems is naturally, through exercise and diet.

Most obstetricians have a recommended diet which they give to their patients. In the second trimester, when your wife is inclined to eat heartily, you should encourage her to follow the diet. The program usually includes eliminating fried or greasy foods, as they are hard to digest and may increase her discomfort; drinking sufficient amounts of liquids, which help to keep stools soft; and adding fresh (raw when possible) fruits and vegetables to increase roughage which stimulates the bowels. If heartburn persists, eating small, frequent meals instead of three big ones is often effective.

Medication

If any of the gastro-intestinal reactions become a real problem, consult your obstetrician. He will not think your wife is making a fuss over nothing, as most pregnant women have the same concerns and he expects these kinds of complaints. If he thinks the situation needs medical attention, he will prescribe one of the many effective products available for treatment of these problems. But in most instances, your doctor will try to solve the problems during pregnancy without unnecessary medications.

No pregnant woman should take medical or chemical products without the express advice of her obstetrician. Many products can have an effect on the unborn child. Your doctor has access to the information which is necessary to make decisions about which medications are considered safe for pregnant women.

Before any medical treatment is needed, you can help your wife by joining her in her diet and a regular program of exercise. You need not be concerned about your wife's suddenly gaining weight by "eating for two." That old wives' tale has caused incalculable problems for expectant mothers. Not only is it unnecessary to eat double portions, it is unhealthy to do so. Excessive weight gain during pregnancy can lead to high blood pressure and considerable strain on the mother's already taxed cardiovascular system.

It is sensible to prevent overweight so that it never becomes a problem. Check with the doctor about what he considers to be an acceptable weight gain. Most obstetricians consider a twenty to twenty-five pound weight gain for the entire pregnancy to be a healthy one for mother and baby. However, if your obstetrician suggests more or less do not argue with him. He is taking into consideration the particular situation which your wife presents and has tailored his advice for her. You can help your wife with this part of her pregnancy by eating what she eats, *without* grumbling. Whether or not the foods would be of your choice, you will find that if you follow the pregnancy diet you will be eating a nutritionally well-balanced diet. You will probably note that you feel healthier yourself.

Most Americans choose to eat a nutritionally poor diet, high in fat and carbohydrate calories. And, although obesity is often a problem in this country, even the obese are often suffering from some degree of malnutrition. It is interesting how many couples who become accustomed to eating the pregnancy diet while expecting, get into the habit of eating properly. This is an excellent habit to develop so you can be a good example for your child to follow as he is growing up.

Program of exercise

Equally as important as proper diet is a regular program of exercise. Physical fitness is a matter of concern at all times of life. Regular exercise improves muscle tone, assists the circulatory system, and helps to burn off some of the excess calories we consume.

The need for exercise does not disappear when a woman becomes pregnant. There is no reason why a woman with an uncomplicated pregnancy cannot continue with her full program of activities. In fact, if she is sedentary, there is good reason to add exercise to her daily routine. Many of the discomforts of pregnancy such as backache or constipation can be alleviated to some extent by exercise.

Your wife should consult the obstetrician if she is interested in doing a particular set of exercises recommended for pregnant women. But even if she objects to formal exercise, you can encourage her throughout pregnancy by joining her in walking. Walking is a nonstrenuous form of exercise that is healthful for both you and your wife. A leisurely walk of an hour or so each day can add stamina to your life.

Later in pregnancy when you both attend classes for childbearing, particular exercises will be introduced that are designed to prepare your wife's muscles for the birth act. For the time being, it is sufficient to engage in just enough activity to maintain a feeling of well-being.

As the pregnancy progresses, you will begin to notice other changes. Toward the end of the second trimester, you will become aware of an uneasiness in your wife. As the baby's presence becomes a reality, the experience of labor and delivery looms big and fearful for most women. As soon as they know of your wife's pregnancy, many women will rush to tell her their own tales of pregnancy and delivery. Many of the experiences of women who were totally unprepared for delivering a baby sound like incredible horror stories.

These stories can only serve to intensify your wife's own fears. Obviously, you cannot lock her up to isolate her from these women and their unfortunate experiences. But you can both begin to prepare yourselves for the coming labor. Much more time will be spent in Chapter two on the details of preparation for childbirth.

Locating educator

The first step towards actual preparation, which you should take near the end of the second trimester, is for you and your wife to locate a teacher, a childbirth educator. For the name of a recognized teacher in your area, contact: The American Society of Childbirth Educators, Inc., 230 Riverside Drive, New York, New York, 10025. The telephone number is (212) 663-3390.

The childbirth educator will schedule you for a series of classes that will prepare *both* of you to actively participate in the labor and delivery of your child. While the classes themselves do not begin until the late seventh or early eighth month, locating a teacher and talking with her about current feelings and learning what can be done now will give your wife enough peace of mind to carry her calmly through until the classes begin. Early registration is a good idea, too, to ensure yourselves a place in the classes within the period close to your delivery date, so that you can complete the course just a short time before delivery.

Classes are made up of several couples expecting within a a few days of each other. They are deliberately small groups to permit the teacher to give each couple personal attention. Yet they are large enough for sharing ideas and experiences within the group. When you let a childbirth educator know that you are interested in attending classes, she will usually send you some literature explaining prepared childbirth and a suggested reading list. These will help the two of you broaden your knowledge and come to classes with enough background to get the most out of them.

THE THIRD TRIMESTER

As you enter the third trimester, you will notice that your wife is experiencing some of the same discomforts that she had earlier in pregnancy. This is related directly to the fact that the growing uterus is so big and heavy with your child that it is causing pressure on the pelvic organs, as well as on the abdominal organs and diaphragm. The obvious results are frequent need to urinate, heartburn, some discomfort when breathing deeply, and in many instances chronic constipation.

The same cues discussed in earlier phases of pregnancy hold for this phase. You can be of great help to your wife by anticipating her discomforts and planning both your lives, for the time being, in ways that will minimize her problems. Just remember, your wife is not more fragile because she is pregnant. She should be encouraged to continue with her usual program of exercise and to add a reasonable amount of walking to her daily activities.

Chronic backache

In addition to the already mentioned discomforts, there are two related symptoms which cause many couples undue alarm. The first symptom is chronic backache. Although backache occurs in most pregnancies, it is understandable and not a sign of

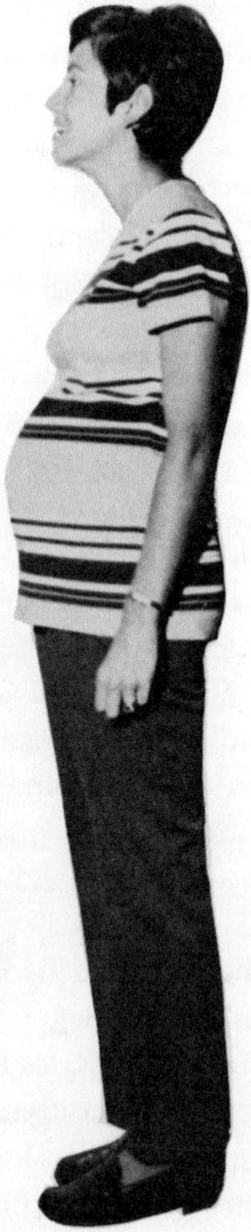

Figure 1

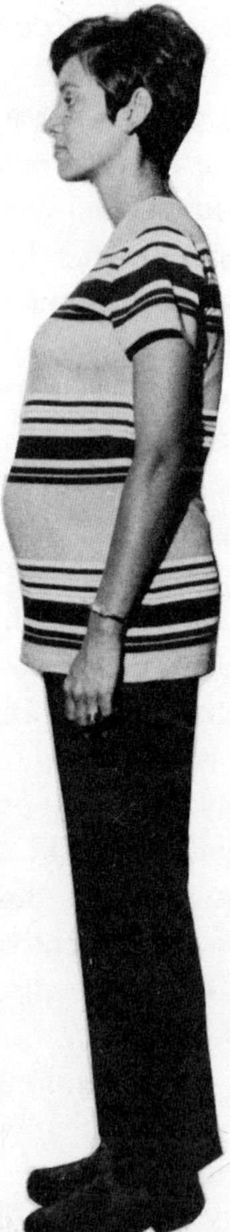

Figure 2

Figure 1. *PREGNANT POSTURE: There is a tendency for a pregnant woman to stand with her shoulders round, belly drooping forward, behind curved out, and head hanging forward in front of chest.*

Figure 2. *GOOD POSTURE: This is in evidence when a person's spine is in alignment. Head should be held high, forcing shoulders back. Hips are rolled forward slightly so buttocks are tucked under.*

internal problems endangering mother or baby. It is rare to find a woman who stands correctly. It is even more rare to find a pregnant woman with good posture. In fact, it is easy to spot a pregnant woman, even if you could not see her big belly. Most pregnant women stand with their feet wide apart, their hips pushed forward, and the upper parts of their bodies leaning backward. It is a sloppy way of responding to the changes of weight distribution.

Initially, it seems like the thing to do to counteract the shift of the center of gravity from mid-pelvis upward with the growth of the pregnant uterus. But this stance creates tremendous tension in the small muscles of the lower back which are not intended to support the additional weight of the gravid (pregnant) uterus. Therefore, the prime way to counteract the backache caused by poor posture is to develop the habit of good posture. This is just as true for you as it is for your wife. Sound easy? If you think it is a snap to "stand up straight," take a good look at yourself in a full length mirror.

Good posture is in evidence when a person's spine is in alignment. This means that if 1) your shoulders are round, or 2) your belly is drooping forward, or 3) your behind is curved out, or 4) your head is hanging forward in front of your chest, you do not have good posture. And any one of these misalignments can cause unpleasant symptoms as muscles are called upon to support parts for which they were not intended. Do you suffer from chronic headaches, upper or lower backache, or chronic fatigue? If you answer yes to any of these questions, you should take a long hard look at your posture.

You can put your spine in proper alignment by thinking of a straight line that passes up from the floor between your legs, through the middle of your pelvis, the middle of your abdominal and chest cavities and comes out the center of the top of your head. You can achieve this alignment by actively setting your body in proper position. Think tall, hold your head as high as

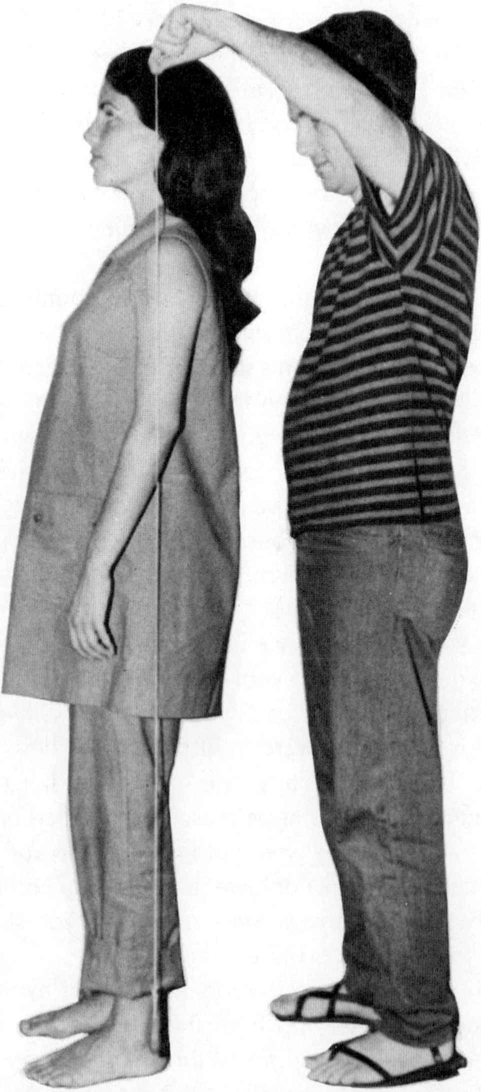

Figure 3. *CHECKING FOR GOOD ALIGNMENT: To check for good bodily alignment, hold a weighted string at ear level and allow it to pass shoulders, hips, knees, and ankles.*

you can. This will force you to bring your shoulders back. Having done this, there only remains for you to roll your hip forward slightly so that your buttocks are tucked under. This is the crucial part of good posture in the pregnant woman as it automatically rolls the abdomen back relieving the lower back muscles of the weight of the uterus.

To maintain good alignment, it is necessary to have a good base. Stand with your feet at least one foot-width apart, with one foot slightly in front of the other. This distributes body weight best on the balls of the feet and along the broad muscles as it should be. If you make good posture a habit, you can not only eliminate backache but also reduce the fatigue that most people experience from standing poorly. This is especially important for your wife whose energy is already taxed by the additional weight she is carrying.

Squatting

There are other ways that good posture can influence your wife while she is pregnant and probably for the rest of her life. One is in bending over. Many of us get into the habit of standing upright and then bending over from the waist. This is not particularly good at any time as it places unnecessary strain on our muscles. But it can be especially harmful for the pregnant woman because when she tips forward, she is suspending the great weight of her pregnancy like a hammock. Not only is this bad for the lower back musculature, but it puts her in an unstable position from which she can easily fall and severly injure herself.

This is so easy to avoid by practicing a little body mechanics. Instead of bending over, squat. With a straight back, bend the legs and hips, resting all the weight on the balls of the feet. This will provide a stable base, as well as a mechanical advantage if something is being lifted. An additional advantage of squatting is that the woman is actually exercising the pelvic floor muscles, the ones she will be using to deliver the baby.

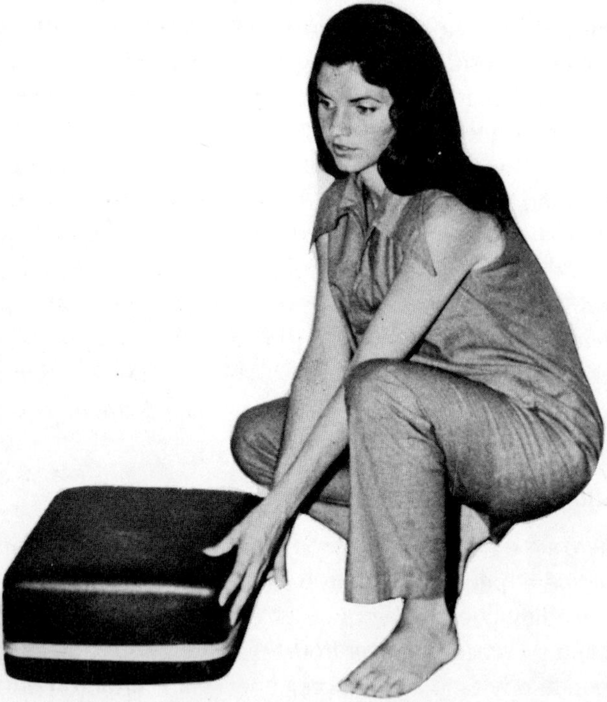

Figure 4. *SQUATTING: It is always better to squat than to bend over. Weight should be on the balls of the feet. Back should be straight.*

Helping your wife achieve good posture should not preclude other husbandly attentions. An offer of a backrub will usually be gratefully received. It gives you a chance to show that you recognize your wife's discomfort and want to help. And, it often provides a relaxing time when the two of you can talk, not of anything in particular, but quietly and together without the strain of day to day problems interfering.

The other symptom often more alarming than backache is a

definite pain, usually described as radiating through the pelvis and down the legs. This can be most alarming to young couples who suspect that the worst has happened. While this does not occur as often as some of the other discomforts, it does happen to enough women to bear mentioning.

This pain cannot cause any permanent damage to mother or baby. The reason for it may be easily explained. It occurs because the uterus is putting pressure on one of the big nerves in the pelvic area. As with any unusual symptom, check with your obstetrician. He will probably tell you that both your wife and baby are fine. It is then up to you to provide care for your wife while she has this problem.

Removing pressure

The main idea behind any care you offer your wife when she has this particular problem is to remove the pressure as much as possible from the pelvic area. For this reason, you will want to encourage your wife to stay in bed. You can make it easier for her by making lying down as comfortable as possible and by having everything she needs within reach.

It is not always simple to make a pregnant woman comfortable in bed. There are the peculiarities of pregnancy to consider. First of all, she is not really sick or an invalid. You should be making suggestions, but please do not make your wife feel like a patient. Consider in planning for your wife's stay in bed what you should do about that big belly. If she is propped up in bed on her back, the weight will still be partially on the nerve. If she lies flat on her back, she may experience tingling in her feet or dizziness because the weight of the baby is sitting right on the big blood vessels surrounding her heart. So, it would be wisest to suggest that your wife find a position on her side. This will put the weight of the baby on the bed.

You can help her get comfortable. Again you will be making

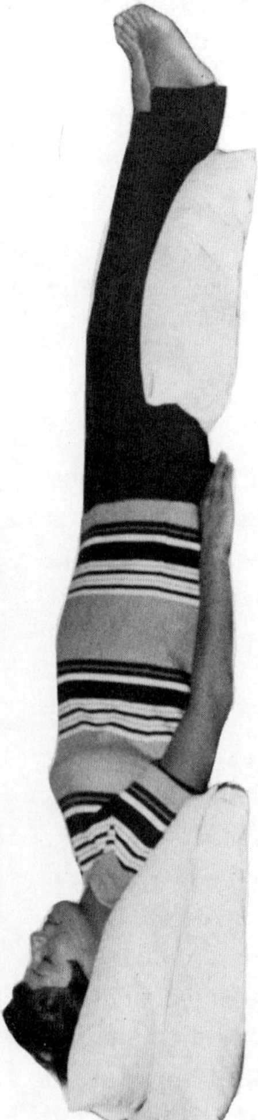

Figure 5

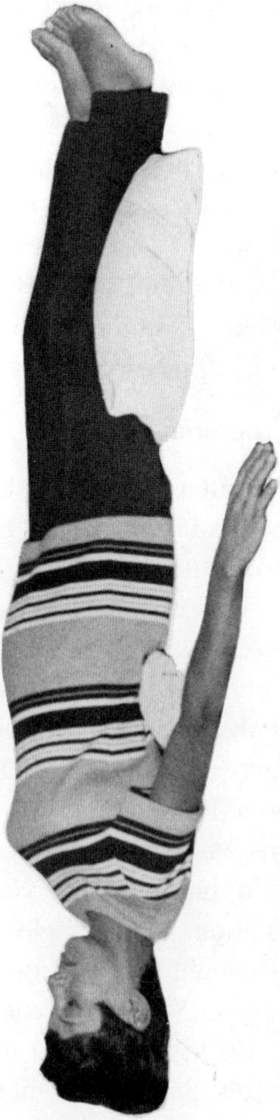

Figure 6

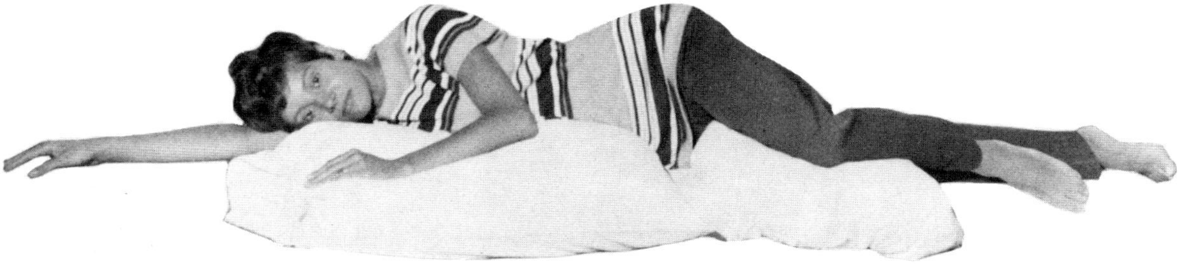

Figure 7

Figure 5. *COMFORT POSITION—RECLINING: This is the basic reclining position. Head and shoulders are supported, and a pillow is under the knees.*

Figure 6. *COMFORT POSITION—RECLINING VARIATION: For the woman who is more comfortable at little or no angle, this variation offers her support for her lower back and legs.*

Figure 7. *COMFORT POSITION—SIDE-LYING: This is a position that many women find comfortable in late pregnancy as well as in labor. The weight of the baby is supported on the bed, and her limbs are supported on pillows.*

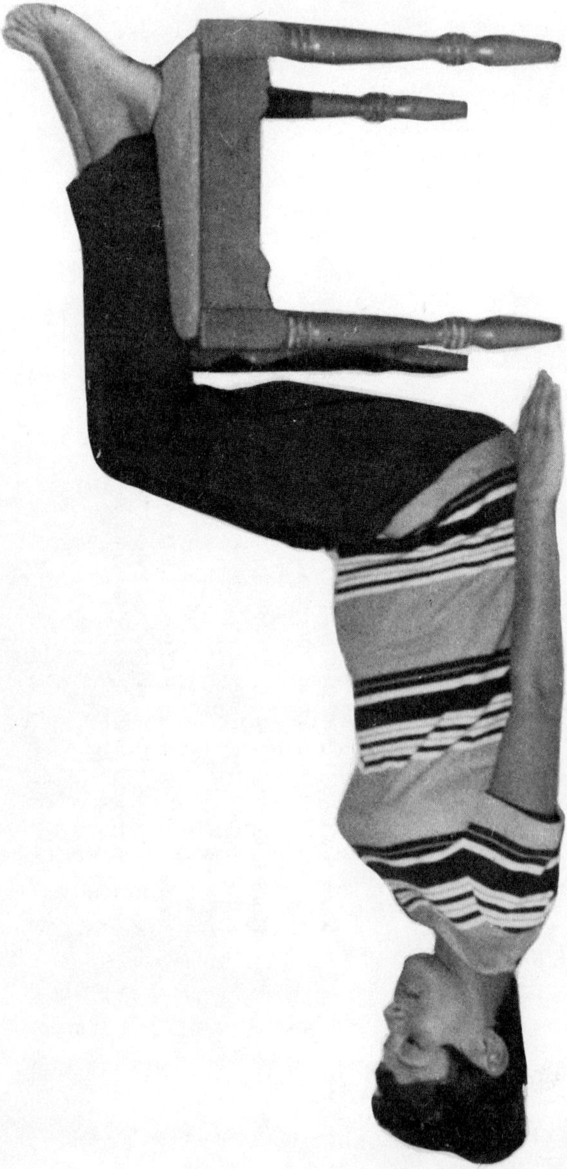

Figure 8. *RELIEVING LOW BACKACHE: When the uterus is putting pressure on one of the big nerves in the pelvic area, resting in this position with one's feet elevated on the base of a chair for ten or fifteen minutes can help relieve the pain.*

logical use of body alignment. To help support her spine in good alignment, you can arrange extra pillows—one under her top arm and one under her top leg. Many women find this a comfortable position for sleeping during the last months of pregnancy anyway. Your wife can roll from side to side and will probably want to change her position frequently.

Keep in mind, she is only in bed for her own comfort. If it becomes tiresome for her, do not insist she stay bedbound. The only person who should decide when and how she should lie is your wife. It is your job to help her stick to her decision by making it as easy as possible for her.

Sexual relations

In talking about the various changes in your relationship that occur because of the inconveniences of pregnancy, you must also consider what changes if any you will need to make about sexual relations between you and your wife during this period.

Although it was considered good medical practice years ago to proscribe intercourse during the last two months of pregnancy, most obstetricians today see no reason for forbidding sex for such a long time. The only real concerns are the comfort and safety of mother and baby. If sexual intercourse causes your wife no distress, there is no reason to abstain. In later pregnancy, most women do experience some discomfort because of the displacement resulting from the pregnant uterus.

You two may have to try new positions until you discover one that is comfortable and pleasurable for you both. If you do not find one that you both enjoy or if intercourse is proscribed for medical reasons, there are other ways that you and your wife can be sensual without actually engaging in intercourse. Mutual fondling can be a satisfactory substitute leading to a climax. As with all sexual activities, this should be acceptable to both partners and engaged in without feelings of guilt.

Other than comfort, safety is the only reason that you would want to stop having sexual relations. If your wife's membranes rupture, there is direct access to the inside of the uterus and the baby. There is a significant possibility of introducing an infection that could endanger your wife's health and the baby's life. For this reason primarily, sexual activity is usually abstained from by most couples during the last two weeks prior to delivery. If you have any questions about your own situation, feel free to discuss them with your obstetrician. Although you may find this a delicate topic to discuss, he is often asked the questions you have in mind.

Finally, the third trimester produces a phenomenon experienced by husband and wife alike. There will be times, especially toward the end of the trimester, when both of you believe that this pregnancy will never end. Although all is normal, the waiting seems interminable.

Because of the guessing game that birthday predictors have to play, your baby can arrive two weeks before or two weeks after the birth date you have been given. Therefore, you should be completely prepared to escort your wife to the hospital at any time from two weeks before the estimated date onward.

By this time you both will have completed your preparation for childbirth course. From the course you will have learned all the basic information about labor and delivery that you will need. If more than two weeks pass from the last class in your course, contact your teacher for a refresher to be sure that your wife is still doing the exercises correctly.

As a husband, there is very little you can actually do to ease the waiting period. However, accompanying your wife's anticipation is the feeling that she is bigger, clumsier, and more unlovely and unloveable than any other woman, especially any other woman who is not nine months pregnant. This is a time when you need to spend a little extra time noticing. Any small attempt to look prettier or act alluring should be immediately noticed by you and complimented.

It will be amazing to you to see how immensely pleased your wife will be to think that there is something about her that you still find attractive. In fact, your compliments will act as a stimulus for her to take the time to look attractive for you. It really works both ways. The more aware you are of the little things, the more attempts she will make to please you.

This is an important time for you to be pleased with each other. You are about to embark on the most exciting experience a couple can share. It will be the hardest work your wife will ever do in her life. You will be doing the most important coaching a husband can do. You two are going to have a baby together. Just as this pregnancy began, an expression of love between husband and wife, so it should end, an experience of sharing and joy in the birth of your baby.

2

Training to Have a Baby

Any good athlete knows that in order to perform at his best, he must be in top physical condition and train those muscles he is going to use for their job. Having a baby is a physical accomplishment every bit as strenuous as running a race or playing a professional sport. Training to have a baby is a process of preparing the mind and the body to work with the forces of labor and delivery. And, just like any other training, it requires a coach.

Anyone familiar with the training situation is well aware of the tremendous importance of the guidance and support of a good coach. This is your role. You, the husband, father of the baby, are part of a team. Your wife is the athlete. Only she can make the effort. Your physician is the manager. He has final say in all matters related to labor and delivery. The nursing staff in the hospital are like trainers, essential in making sure that your wife and baby remain in the best physical condition throughout.

But you are the coach. You can help your wife all along the way. You will be calling on your knowledge of her, on your understanding of the process of labor and delivery, on your ability to predict what she should be doing, and on all your strength as a man and a husband to help her have your baby in the best way possible for herself, for the baby, and for you. For this reason, you and your wife have to go into a training period. You both must learn everything you can about labor and delivery. Your wife needs to know so she will be able to understand what she is experiencing. You need to know so that you will be able to offer the best guidance for coping at any point in labor.

PPM PHILOSOPHY

Psychoprophylaxis is a long, unwieldy name that refers to the prevention (prophylaxis) of mental or emotional (psycho) trauma experienced by most unprepared women during the process of childbearing. Because we learn that having a baby is a painful experience, we expect it to be so. This belief coupled with lack of factual information detailing a step by step description of labor and delivery leaves the unprepared woman without any understanding of what has happened or what she can expect to happen. All she knows is what she feels. And what she has learned to expect to feel—pain.

Obstetrics has dealt with this situation by blotting out the experience through the use of medication. However, this has not been satisfactory to many intelligent women who are left with a void in their memories. All they remember is the pain and loss of control they experienced. This leaves the majority of these women with a sense of having failed somehow at a time when they know they should be happy and proud of all that they have accomplished. All around it is a negative experience. The poor husband, if he sees his wife in labor at all, feels helpless and even guilty about placing his wife in a painful, uncontrolled situation. He too starts out on a new life with a bad feeling that could have been avoided.

Labor need not be as painful as we have learned it is supposed to be. Labor is, as it is named, hard physical work. It is the hardest work a woman will do in her whole life. But it should result in a job that is accomplished with all the feelings that go along with achievement. For this, we modern, civilized people must be specially prepared.

Dick-Read theory

The theory explaining pain in childbirth that is now generally accepted by educators was first described by the English obstetrician Dr. Grantly Dick-Read. Dr. Dick-Read believed that the pain experienced in childbirth is a result of muscular tension. He also believed that most women were so ignorant about their bodies and childbirth in general that when they arrived at the hospital in labor, they were paralyzed with fear. The fear resulted in generalized muscular tension which served to intensify the sensations of the labor contractions. The more intense labor became the more fearful and tense the women grew. This fear-tension-pain cycle snowballs for the untrained woman into an experience of unrelenting, painful contractions that many women retell as their own personal horror stories.

A woman's ignorance is her own worst enemy. Recognizing this, Dr. Dick-Read developed a program of training that served to de-educate women about childbearing. Under his guidance, women were encouraged to abandon superstitions and to learn the facts about the process of labor and delivery. As part of this type of training, known as the Read method, the doctor encouraged his patients to relax totally during a labor contraction, as well as between contractions. It required focusing all mental energies on relaxation. Because this method also placed emphasis on the elimination of medication for childbirth, it became known popularly as "natural childbirth."

The method seemed to work very well under the artful guidance of Dr. Dick-Read. However, when brought to this country, the Read method underwent many changes in the hands of self-appointed teachers who found that the American personality had difficulty accepting the role of passivity that the method advocates. The Read method declined in use in this country without the personal charisma of Dr. Grantly Dick-Read. But his theory of the fear-tension-pain cycle still serves as a strong basis for most programs educating couples for childbirth.

It is unfortunate that in America we the public are so often the victims of our great scientific advancement. Our advancement in the use of anesthesia has resulted in its indiscriminate use in labor and delivery, and, as a consequence, many couples have been cheated of the opportunity to participate actively in the birth of their children.

This country was the first to have safe anesthesia, carefully administered by qualified anesthesiologists. As a result, after World War II it became popular to offer women "painless childbirth." The growth of anesthesia in labor and delivery was phenomenal. This is the only country that uses anesthesia for childbirth when it is *not* absolutely necessary. Because the long-range effects of anesthesia on the unborn child and his development have never clearly been determined, there really was never any strong movement to return to a more sensible prescription of anesthesia until the "natural childbirth" movement spearheaded by the Read method.

Establishing ASPO

However, a high percentage of these women who were attempting to use the Read method finally resorted to anesthesia. Therefore, their obstetricians were not challenged in their indiscriminate use of anesthesia. Not, that is, until the efforts of the late Marjorie Karmel brought to the general public the idea of actively participating in childbirth.

Mrs. Karmel had the opportunity to have a baby in France using the psychoprophylactic method under the guidance of

Dr. Fernand Lamaze. She returned to this country bringing the method with her. It was very difficult to gain wide acceptance by the medical professions, although she quickly found supporters among mothers like herself. Finally, Mrs. Karmel and Elisabeth Bing, R.P.T., a pioneer in teaching the method in this country, managed to motivate a handful of forward-looking obstetricians to establish The American Society for Psychoprophylaxis in Obstetrics, the first medical society devoted to this method in the United States. Later expanded to include teacher and parent members, ASPO has made the psychoprophylactic method (PPM) available to thousands of couples across America.

Because it offers husbands and wives the opportunity to participate actively in the birth of their child, this method of preparation for labor and delivery has rapidly spread. As taught here today, PPM differs from the experience Mrs. Karmel had in France in the fifties.

At that time, women attended classes with a monitrice, or female coach. The monitrice provided training in conjunction with class preparation provided by the physician. It was the monitrice who attended the woman in labor. The husband, if he was present at all, was an observer.

This is not the situation today. American proponents of PPM recognized the advantages of the husband participating. It is far more valuable for a husband and wife to work together than to introduce another professional into the stressful situation of labor and delivery. Therefore, preparation for childbirth in the psychoprophylactic method is taught in this country as a family experience. Both partners are encouraged to attend classes.

Most husbands step into the first class somewhat hesitantly and in the majority of cases skeptically. Many feel that they have only come along to humor a pregnant wife. You may have some of these feelings yourself, especially if you have been talking to some of your less fortunate buddies who cannot understand why you are "invading a woman's world." Your uneasiness will last just until you step through the door and find yourself in a room with several other pregnant couples.

You are all in the same boat together. Each of you will be delivering at about the same time. And each of you will be sharing the six sessions preparing for the important job ahead of you. This will probably be the first time you can talk to other men who really understand what you want because they are seeking the same thing for themselves and their wives. You will be reassured when you start to talk among yourselves and find out just how much you have in common.

Education is the primary concern of PPM classes. In order for you to understand the techniques of PPM training, an overall view of the labor and delivery processes is necessary.

OVERALL VIEW OF LABOR

One should know that labor is a process. Once it has begun, it moves ahead in a predictable pattern. The force of labor is muscular activity called contractions. A contraction is a tightening and shortening of the uterine muscles for the purpose of moving the baby down and out of the vagina. There is a portal that connects the uterus and the vagina, which is called the cervix. The cervix is long and thick and closed when labor begins. It has served to protect the baby from the outside world all during the pregnancy. But it must become thin (efface) and open up (dilate) to allow the baby to be born.

At the beginning of labor, the cervix resembles a jug neck and must open to resemble a mayonnaise jar. The distance of opening is estimated when the doctor examines your wife internally. He may express the dilatation in terms of centimeters, from zero to ten; or he may express the dilatation in terms of fingers, from zero to five.

The terms may be used interchangeably, and usage really

depends on which school of medicine your physician attended. But you should be aware that two centimeters are equal to one finger so that if during labor you hear different terms being used you will know that your wife is still making progress. Once the cervix is fully dilated to ten centimeters, the baby is ready to move out of the uterus and make the final maneuvers in being born.

Beginning labor

Labor can begin in a number of ways. The first sign that some women experience is the rupturing of their membranes. A woman may have a sudden gush of clear, odorless fluid or a steady trickle that she cannot control. Either event is usually a surprise as the membrane itself has no nerve endings and your wife may have no warning that this is about to happen.

Other women begin labor without any change in their membranes. For these women the first indications are mild, barely perceptible contractions. To try to comprehend what this feels like, make a fist. The muscles in your forearm are contracting. This sensation is not particularly painful although you are aware that your forearm is tightened. The woman in early labor may experience a similar sensation as a tightening across her abdomen. Or she may experience a low backache. The only difference is that you can voluntarily start and stop the contraction of your forearm. And, in fact, you would when you felt the muscles getting tired.

The process of labor cannot voluntarily be turned off. So, it will be one of your jobs to see that your wife conserves as much of her energy as possible to prevent fatigue. Some women have no sensation at all during this early, preliminary period of labor. However, no matter what the signs you notice, there is work going on inside your wife. If this is your first baby, labor may begin as early as two weeks before the due date. The cervix is beginning to thin down, or efface. Your wife will probably get this kind of report from the doctor when she goes for her checkup a week or two before you expect the baby.

As you and your wife become aware of early labor, you will be able to distinguish the contractions. They begin in the low back and radiate forward around the lower abdomen. As labor progresses, the contractions will become closer together, last longer, and the sensation will be stronger. This is still a time for you and your wife to rest. The hard work lies ahead.

Your doctor will probably have you bring your wife to the hospital when the contractions are coming at about five minute intervals. He may ask you to come in sooner if he thinks you might have problems with transportation or if your wife's membranes have been ruptured for more than twenty-four hours. The latter is an uncommon occurrence which can result in severe infection for mother and baby. It is a medical judgment, and if the doctor asks you to bring her in earlier than you had planned, trust his judgment and bring her without an argument. If you have been open with him, there should be no problem regardless of when you arrive at the hospital.

By the time your wife is in a labor room in the hospital, you two will probably be working together on the techniques you have been practicing. Labor will continue to progress. The contractions will be following a pattern, lasting almost a minute and fairly strong. The cervix will be dilating. A doctor will examine your wife at regular intervals and keep you informed of the progress. You may have to ask him each time.

Transition

The hardest part of labor occurs just before the cervix is completely dilated. The baby is moving down with each contraction resulting in considerable rectal pressure and causing the urge to push. You and your wife will have to work hard during this period, called transition, to keep her from pushing. If she pushes too soon, it can cause what little bit of cervix is left to become swollen and prolong this difficult period of labor. Although this is the most difficult period, it is the shortest. Most couples can get through transition by using the techniques and by reminding each other that the baby will soon be born.

Once the cervix is completely dilated, your wife will be given permission to push. Your wife, who only a few minutes before would have gladly chucked the whole thing, suddenly has renewed energy and feels so much better since she is able to do something positive. The baby could be born if she were completely unconscious. But she can use her abdominal and chest muscles to assist the uterus and in that way shorten the delivery stage. Even though this is strenuous physical exercise, most women find pushing a tremendous relief. And, by this time, you both know the baby is soon to born.

In your preparation classes, you will learn what you both can do at each point in labor and delivery. Even though you attend the same classes, you must remember that you and your wife will be seeing things from a different perspective. She will be involved in learning as a participant. You will be learning as her coach. You must never forget that you have an objectivity that she as a woman about to be in labor can never have. It is for this reason that you should make every effort to attend all of the classes. In this way, you will have the best preparation to act as coach both in the practice sessions at home and in actual labor.

HOW PPM OPERATES

Psychoprophylaxis preparation is a method which combines selective neuro-muscular control and complex patterns of deliberate, coordinated breathing techniques. In labor, the trained woman concentrates on consciously relaxing all of her body that is not involved in the contraction and on breathing in direct response to the sensation that she perceives with the contraction.

This combination of physical and mental activity replaces the fear-tension-pain cycle with a cycle of knowledge-relaxation-control. She is very busy, just as an athlete is busy during the height of a play. He does not feel a bad bruise until the play is over. It is the same with the trained woman. She is so occupied with the business of concentrating that she is not aware of painful sensations during a contraction.

This method does not promise a totally painless childbirth. Pain is subjective, meaning different things to different people depending on how they perceive it in a given situation. The perception of pain is in part related to the individual's threshold of pain, or the point at which a sensation feels painful. One person feels severe pain in a situation where another might interpret the sensation as only hurting a little. This has to do with the individual's physical and emotional condition, as well as the circumstances in which he is at the moment.

In prepared childbirth, the sensations of labor are reduced to a tolerable, controllable level. In fact, many trained women report only having perceived sensations of pressure or discomfort. By preparing themselves ahead of time, they have equipped their minds to understand the process of labor. What begins for most women as sensations of pressure or stretching remains that way for the trained woman.

But as with any accomplishment, you get out of it what you put into it. No athlete can expect to perform at his best unless he thoroughly knows all the maneuvers of his sport and practices to keep in peak condition. So it is with the woman in labor. She must know what she can do to help herself at any point in labor. As her coach you must know, too. She must practice regularly right up to the day she delivers. It is imperative that you as her coach practice with her everyday. You must know what your wife is supposed to be doing. That alone is not enough however.

You must also know what she looks like when she is doing her exercises. Practicing together while at home gives you the opportunity to learn what to look for—tension, sloppy technique irritability—while it is still only practice. At home, you are both relaxed. You can perfect the techniques you learn in class. Your wife will become accustomed to responding to your verbal cues. This is vital.

Labor is a time of stress, physically and emotionally. By training, it is hoped that your wife will respond automatically to the labor sensations within her body. As labor progresses, the response may need the prompting of your verbal cues. A simple reminder like "Relax your legs, honey" can often make the difference between conserving stamina and early fatigue. This is one of your most important jobs as labor coach.

Fatigue is the biggest enemy of physical activity. Fatigue results in slowed reflexes and muscular irritability. More important, fatigue leads to depression and emotional irritability. It will definitely interfere with your wife's ability to retain control. Therefore, as her coach, you must practice looking for signs of tension—tight neck, tensed arms or legs, frowning—almost from the beginning of your sessions at home together. Practice telling her to relax the tense part or gently touch it as you speak. In this way, you will be developing between yourselves a system of communication that will work automatically during labor.

This may sound like a lot of work; it is! No physical skills are learned by reading and watching alone. Labor is not a spectator sport. Labor requires active participation if it is going to be a meaningful and shared experience. However, because practice does require so much attention, it is suggested that the course be taken in the last two months of pregnancy. This allows you to work closely together to learn and perfect your skills so that you and your wife will be at peak performance at the time labor begins. If you begin classes much earlier than that, you will find that your enthusiasm and diligence decline. Not being in top shape, you cheat yourselves. If you start your classes later than six weeks before your due date, chances are you will not finish the course.

Talk about exercises often conjures up a mental picture of Mr. America hoisting a barbell. In preparing for childbirth, exercises are designed to improve body tone, to promote comfort, and to develop the ability to selectively relax groups of muscles while others are working. Most people in the civilized world are not physically fit for labor or any other prolonged strenuous activity. Because it is not prudent to entertain a body-building course during pregnancy, the best thing is to prepare those muscles which will have to work the hardest during labor and delivery.

TAILOR-SITTING EXERCISES

Probably the easiest exercise of all is tailor-sitting. That is right. Tailor-sitting is an exercise. By sitting on a flat surface with ankles crossed and brought close to the body with thighs close to the floor, the lower back is curved. These small muscles of the lumbo-sacral area are relaxed and the strain of the increased weight of the pregnant uterus is temporarily shifted to other muscles for support. This is also a good way to relieve backache. Many women assume tailor-sitting because it is so comfortable. In this position, two exercises, variations of tailor-sitting, can be done to build body stamina and to prepare the muscles of the upper body and the abdomen and legs.

The first variation is designed to expand the chest muscles and make the woman aware of those groups of muscles she uses in breathing. Although only a preliminary exercise, it is extremely important because of the breathing techniques she will be learning for coping with labor. She must be aware of the muscles so that she can use them most effectively.

Therefore, in the tailor-sitting position, the first variation will begin by imagining a bar a full arm's length above the head. Then with a straight spine, looking straight ahead, reach up as if to grasp the bar, first with one arm then with the other. Each time the arm reaches inhale; exhale when the arm relaxes. Alternate

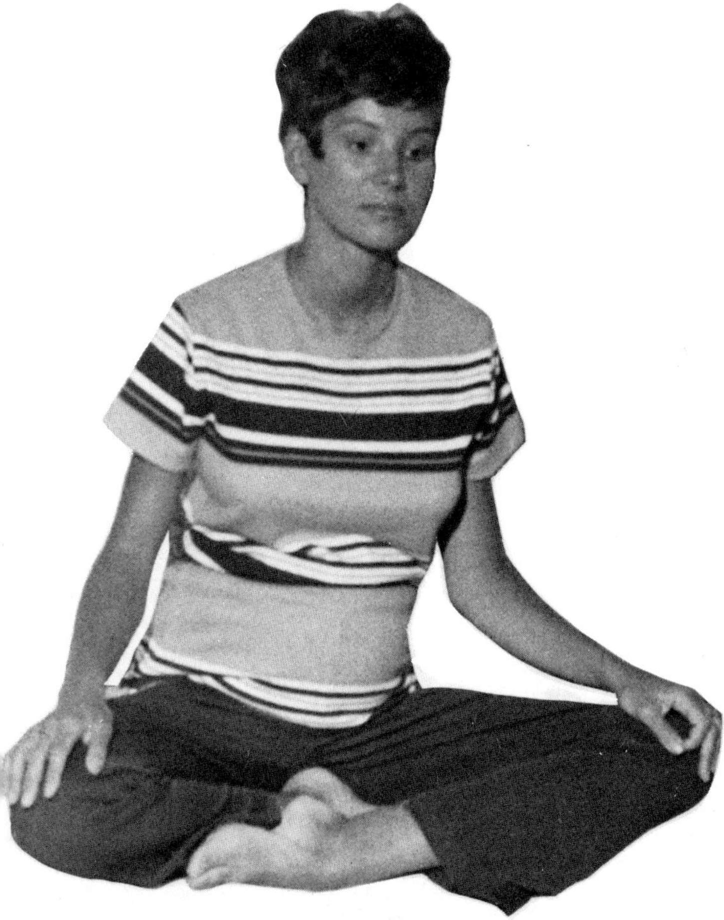

Figure 9. *TAILOR SITTING: Sit on a flat surface with ankles crossed and brought close to the floor. Lower back is curved. Small muscles of the lumbo-sacral areas are relaxed. Weight of pregnant uterus is shifted to other muscles for support.*

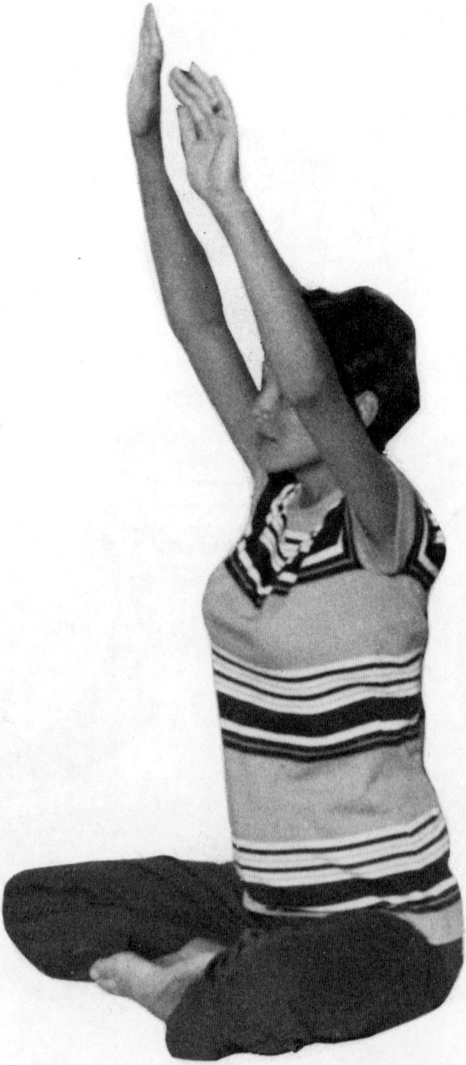

Figure 10. *TAILOR REACH: Imagine a bar a full arm's length above the head. With a straight spine and looking straight ahead, reach up as if to grasp the bar, first with one arm, then with the other. As arm reaches, inhale. As it relaxes, exhale. Alternate arms ten times.*

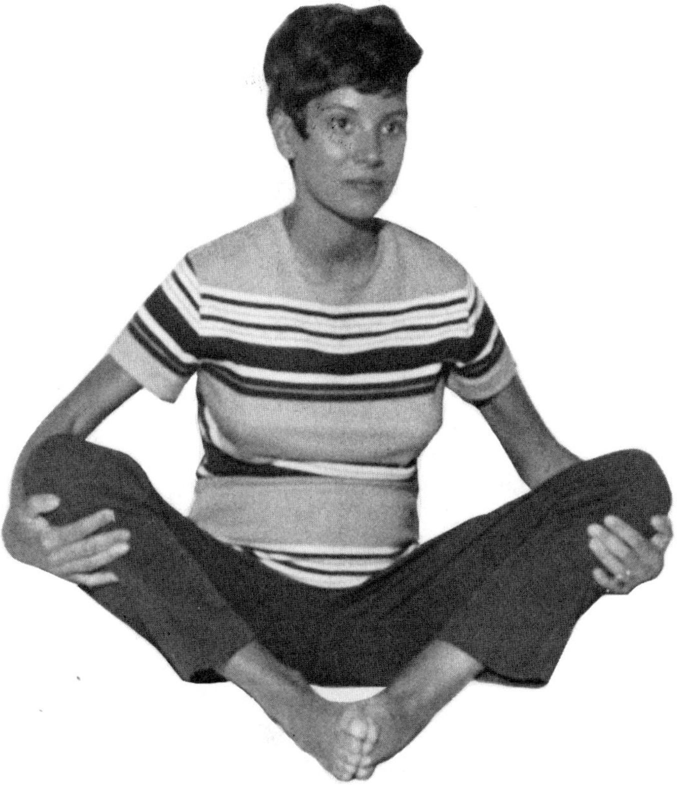

Figure 11. *TAILOR PRESS: Ankles should be uncrossed and soles of feet pressed together as close to the body as comfortable. Palm of hand should be placed under each knee. As deep breath is exhaled, press knees down on palms of hands.*

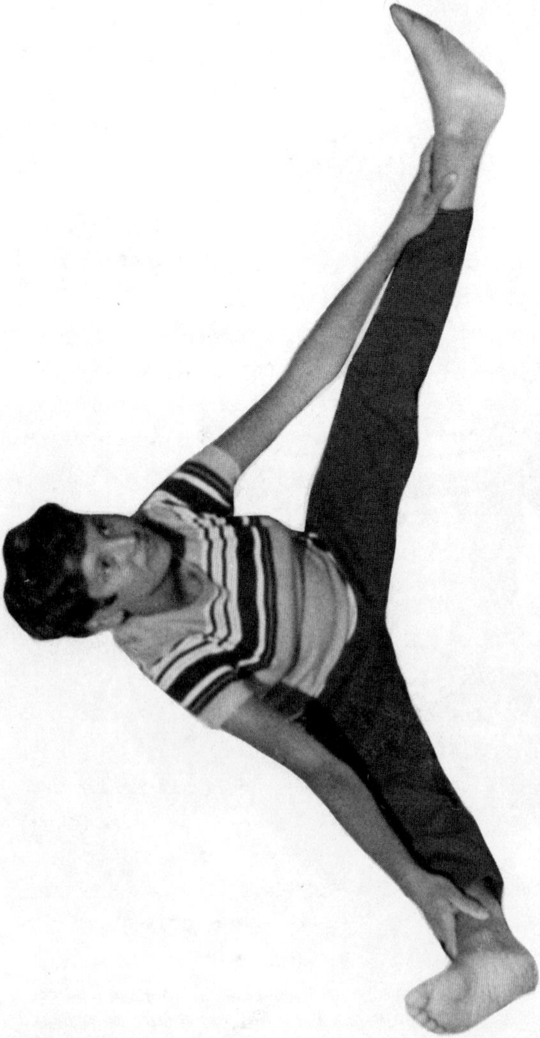

Figure 12. TAILOR STRETCH: *Sitting with legs stretched out in front, let feet rotate a little outward. Extend arms and keeping back straight, reach toward toes. Inhale . . . relax; exhale . . . reach. This is an alternate exercise for the woman who does not feel the muscles on the inside of her thighs working when she is doing the tailor press.*

arms for a total of ten times. Think while doing this exercise, "Which muscles are working and which are relaxed?" This exercise is also a good one for stretching the upper back muscles; it feels good.

The second variation that is begun in the tailor-sitting position is designed to increase the stamina in the thigh muscles, very important for the delivery stage. Ankles should be uncrossed and soles of feet pressed together. Feet should be as close to the body as they can comfortably be held. The palm of the hand should be placed under each knee. To combine the exercise with breathing, a breath should be inhaled, and as it is exhaled, the knees should press down on the palms of the hands.

The rhythm should be: inhale . . . relax, exhale . . . press, inhale . . . relax, exhale . . . press. This exercise should be done *slowly* and *rhythmically* for a total of ten times.

If your wife finds that this exercise is too easy or does not feel the muscles on the inside of her thighs working, there is an alternate exercise that she can do. Sitting with legs stretched out in front of her, letting the feet rotate a little outward, she can extend her arms and with a straight back reach toward her toes. The breathing sequence is the same. Inhale . . . relax; exhale . . . reach. She will feel this in her thighs as a stretching sensation if she is doing it correctly.

Perineal tightening

An exercise that can actually be done in any position but that should be practiced with the tailor-sitting to insure regularity, is the perineal tightening, or Kegel exercise. The perineum is that small patch of flesh that extends between the vagina and the rectum. In some cultures, women's normal work patterns include crouching for long periods, which encourages the perineal muscles to work. In our sedentary society, women consider such activities ungraceful and avoid using the muscles. As a result, our women must make a special effort to get the perineal muscles in top shape to do their job at delivery. This is the intention of the perineal tightening exercise, which sounds much more complicated than it is.

To understand which muscles are involved, imagine you are driving on a parkway with many miles between exits. You have just passed an exit. Suddenly you discover that you need to urinate, urgently. Tighten all the muscles you would have to until you reach the next exit.

Although external genitalia are so obviously different in men and women, the internal musculature is similar enough for you to understand this maneuver. The reason this is emphasized for you here is that in the practice sessions with your wife you have a job with this exercise. No, you will not be expected to check which muscles are contracted. Your job is to observe your wife's overall body tension. With perineal tightening, she will be using muscles that for most women have never been consciously, voluntarily contracted. She will be concentrating hard. The normal tendency is to tense the rest of the body, especially the shoulders, head, and neck. Your job is to watch for signs of tension and remind her to relax. This is excellent practice for you as it is one of your most important jobs in actual labor.

DISCRIMINATE ACTIVITIES

Tension and relaxation are the keys to using PPM. Until now, we have been talking about exercises that prepare the body. Peripherally mentioned was that some exercises create an awareness of muscular use. There is a definite exercise program intended to prepare your wife for deliberate, controlled relaxation in labor. It is a series of discriminate muscular activities that you both must practice and master together.

The importance of this series of exercises is the conditioning of the body to respond to tension in one group of muscles by complete relaxation of all other muscles in the body. This prepares for the situation in labor when the goal during each uterine contraction is relaxation. Of all the exercises you practice together, this set is probably the most important. For, by conditioning your wife's body to relax automatically with muscular tension as the stimulus, you will be helping her to work with her labor and to conserve the precious energy that will allow her to cope with and to control her own body.

Your role during these practice sessions is to learn your wife's particular reactions to tension, to look for hidden tensions, and to develop a system of verbal cues that your wife will learn to respond to automatically. It is the automatic response that is essential to the labor situation.

Controlled relaxation should be practiced initially in a semi-reclining position, with a pillow under your wife's shoulders and knees so that she is comfortable. Later as the two of you gain precision, the position should be modified to include sitting and side-lying so that she will be able to relax in whatever position she finds comfortable in labor.

Meanwhile, for the practice sessions she will probably be most comfortable if you place two pillows behind her back so that she is resting comfortably at approximately a forty-five degree angle. Another pillow should be placed under her knees to relieve any strain in the muscles of her lower abdomen. With your wife in this position, you are ready to begin practice of controlled relaxation.

To create an awareness of body tension, there is a preliminary routine that should precede each set of controlled relaxation practice sessions. During the preliminary routine it is especially important for you to observe your wife closely so that you can learn what she looks like when she is deliberately tensing different parts of her body and when she then consciously relaxes.

CONTROLLED RELAXATION - PRELIMINARY ROUTINE

	Husband's Cues	Wife's Reactions	What to look for
1)	"Stretch legs down"	Push down through legs; keeping foot flexed, push heel as far as possible	Tight muscles the length of the leg; foot held tightly
	"Relax"	Let legs flop	Contract loose muscles with those tense during exercise
2)	"Stretch spine"	Pull top of spine up while pushing the lower portion down	Tension throughout torso, will probably include shoulders and possibly arms and legs
	"Relax"	Let spine fall back against pillows	Body loses tension; note how she looks when relaxed
3)	"Contract buttocks"	Tighten the muscles of the buttocks	Body will be slightly raised in the area of the lower back as tight buttocks create a bridge
	"Relax"	Let all muscles go allowing back to fall back on pillows	Back will rest on support—no space visible under lower spine
4)	"Stretch arms"	Push down through arms, through palms of hands; extend fingers reaching as far as possible without lifting shoulders	Tension along arms, and in shoulders; fingers tense

Husband's Cues	Wife's Reactions	What to look for
"Relax"	Allow arms to flop	Arms resting loosely at side; fingers slightly curled in repose
5) "Shrug shoulders"	Bring shoulders as high as possible beside head without lifting them off pillows	Shoulders tense, neck tense may be able to see blood vessels standing out; head held rigidly
"Relax"	Let shoulders flop back to normal	All parts rest against support
6) "Frown"	Make a face and hold as tightly as possible	Facial muscles taut; worried look; head rigid; neck tense
"Relax"	Let your face return to normal	Face in repose; head resting on pillow

During the preliminary routine, you have an opportunity to observe how different parts of your wife's body—arms, legs, face, neck—look when she is tense. This is important information to you as a coach, not only for the practice sessions but also for actual labor. She will be much too busy trying to carry out the techniques as she has learned them to be fully aware of unnecessary tension. This is your job. You must carefully look for all the tension areas that you saw in the preliminary routine.

In practice, you and your wife will work out a system of either verbal cues such as "Relax your left arm" or tactile cues such as stroking a tense left arm. It is during the controlled relaxation practice that you will develop this system. The actual exercises of controlled relaxation are for the purpose of developing an automatic response in your wife. In labor you will not be using the exact exercises that you practice. But you will be depending on the learned relaxation response. For this you must develop expertise in the area of relaxation. Your wife must learn that in labor she must use only those muscles absolutely necessary during a contraction.

Incidentally, this is a principle we could all learn. One reason most urbanized people are short of energy and stamina is that they are constantly tense. Make a conscious attempt to use only those muscles necessary for any activity whether it is sitting, walking, or talking on a telephone. You will be amazed if you can relax enough to do it. You will be able to do more physically. And you will find that you can be more relaxed about the emotional pressures of daily living. Relax and live longer.

In labor, your wife will have no control over the rhythmic, involuntary contractions of the uterus. Because you both understand the progress of labor, you will be able to approximate the interval and duration of the contraction. The breathing techniques, to be discussed in detail later, will give your wife a tool with which to cope with the contraction. But she cannot stop or start a contraction at will. For that reason, in practicing the controlled relaxation you will give the verbal cues. You will need to indicate when to begin contracting, which muscles to contract, and when to relax. While your wife contracts the specified muscles, she must concentrate on keeping all other parts of her body relaxed. To do this, she must attempt to forget about the contracted part and deliberately think about relaxing all the others.

One aid to concentrating is focusing the eyes on an unmoving object, trying to exclude all else that might be distracting. Some women try to eliminate this step, saying that they can concentrate better with their eyes closed. This is a fallacy. With the eyes closed, the mind tends to wander away from the business of concentrating, and in labor this can lead to loss of control.

In the practice session, your major job will be checking for relaxation. You will also use this coach's tool when your wife is in labor. As you practice, you will be able to quickly observe her state of relaxation or tension. In the beginning you should work with a checklist.

Checking relaxation

First, observe your wife's overall appearance. Is she frowning? Are her fingers on the untensed hand tightly curled or clenched? Are the toes of her untensed foot flexed? Do her neck or shoulders look rigid?

To check for relaxation while your wife is contracting an arm or leg or combination, slide your hand into the hand of her relaxed arm, as if you were going to shake hands. Take hold of her hand and lift the arm up. All of its weight should hang from your hand. As you hold her hand, gently swing the arm back and forth. When she is relaxed, you will be able to do this very easily and observe the arm swinging freely from the shoulder. But this does take concentration and practice on her part.

You will find that in the beginning she will offer you her hand, or grasp your hand when you take hold of hers, or lift her arm with you. These are natural reactions and will take some effort to overcome. Your job is to recognize these reactions and say, "Relax this arm. Let it hang from my hand." Hold the hand firmly and gently rock the arm back and forth. Repeat the words and the rocking, and you will find that your wife will be able to relax her arm.

To check the relaxed leg, you place both hands gently behind the knee and lift the leg slightly and allow it to fall back on the pillow. If it is relaxed, the heel of the foot will slide along the floor as you lift the knee. If it is tense, the leg will be stiff and hard to move. You will probably find this most often when the other leg is contracted. Again, use the verbal as well as tactile cues. Say "Relax this leg" and check it again, repeating until it

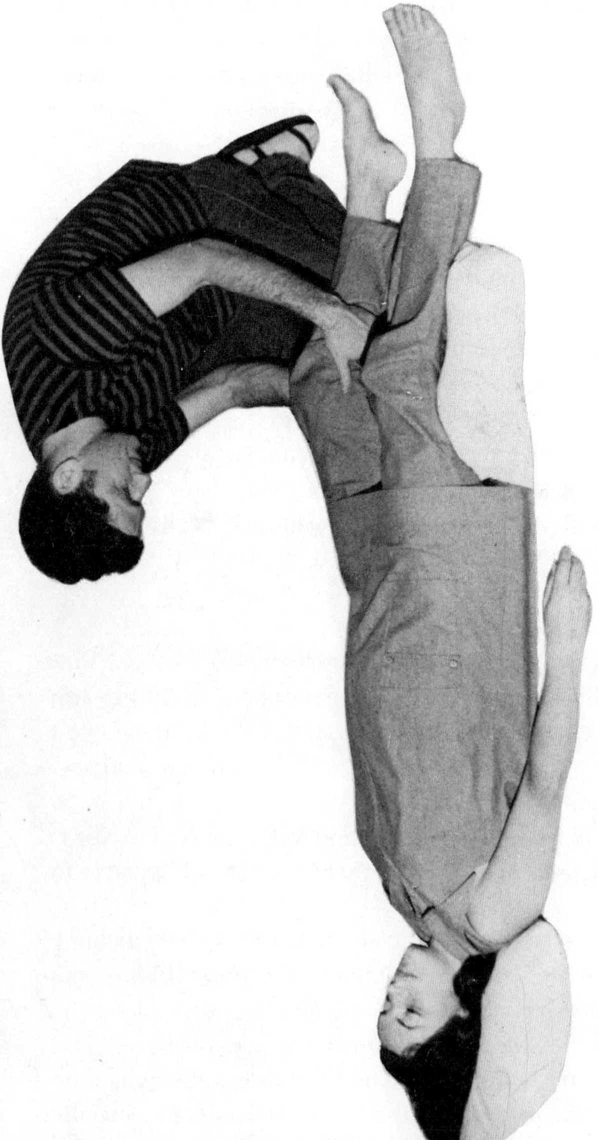

Figure 13. *CHECKING FOR RELAXATION: The coach should check for tension in all parts that are not being deliberately tightened for the exercise.*

is relaxed or until you think that you two should stop the exercise.

It is extremely important that you remember to tell your wife. to relax after each contraction. If you are to develop a pattern where she can relax completely on your cue, you must always provide the cue. Do not become so engrossed in checking her that you forget to give her the "relax" direction. Remember, your goal is cooperation in labor. You want your cues to be so deeply set that she will respond to them automatically, without conscious thought when she is actually in labor. Most labor contractions last for less than a full minute. Your controlled relaxation practice should not be longer than a minute for any sequence.

CONTROLLED RELAXATION PRACTICE

	Husband's cue	Wife's reaction	What to look for
1)	"Contract right arm"	Make a fist of right hand and raise a few inches	Check to see if wife has eyes focused; check left arm and both legs; give direction to relax
	"Relax"	Arm should drop back on support	Check to see that arm drops and is not consciously lowered
2)	"Contract left arm"	Same as for right arm	Same as for right arm
	"Relax"		
3)	"Contract left leg"	Pull toes of foot as close to body as possible (flex foot); tighten muscles of leg as if it were to be raised	Check for eye focus; check both arms and right leg—it is especially difficult in the beginning to tense one leg and relax the other; check to see if buttocks are tense (hard)

	Husband's Cues	Wife's Reactions	What to look for
	"Relax"	Leg should go limp	Check leg for relaxation before going on
4)	"Contract both arms"	Tighten both fists	Check for tension in neck and face; check legs
	"Relax"	Both arms should drop	Same as with one arm; both should drop and not be lowered
5)	"Contract both legs"	Flex both feet	Check both arms and head and neck for tension
	"Relax"	Both legs should go limp	Check legs for relaxation
6)	"Contract both shoulders"	Shrug shoulders	Check hands and both legs; observe face for tension
	"Relax"	Let shoulders return to normal position	Check neck for tension

POINTS TO REMEMBER

You are working together. As a coach, it is your responsibility to see that your wife remains motivated. People learn best when they feel that they are accomplishing something. Be sure to tell her what she is doing well *before* you launch into what she has not been doing properly. As you practice more and more, you will find that there is less to be improved. But in the beginning, especially, you must be aware of your own criticisms. Avoid saying things like "That was all wrong." No matter how good your intentions or how lovingly you say it, that kind of criticism can turn your sessions into competitions.

You and your wife must be working toward a time when you will act together as a precision team. She needs you. So direct your efforts at this point toward building up her confidence in you as her coach. She is working hard in these practice sessions. Probably she is not aware of what she is actually doing, only of what she is trying to do. You, on the other hand, are able to see exactly what she is doing and know what it should be. But before you tell her, be sure to notice what she is doing well, even if it is only focusing her eyes.

Complex combinations

After your wife has mastered contracting one limb at a time (this usually occurs by about the second practice session), you should move ahead to more complex combinations. Even if she has not completely mastered the first set, by moving ahead she will find that the first set is easier to do than she thought. The purpose of these exercises is to selectively relax those muscles not actually doing work. You will be looking for the same points of tension and relaxation as with the simpler exercises. The only real change is in the cues you give your wife. You can use any combination and should vary them to challenge her ability to concentrate. Some cues that you might use are:

Contract left arm, right leg . . . relax. Contract left arm, left leg . . . relax. Contract right arm, left leg . . . relax. Contract left arm, right leg . . . relax. Contract both legs, make a face . . . relax.

Over the years, husbands have been ingenious in inventing combinations. As you practice with your wife, you will find that as she gains more skill at relaxing, you can speed up the directions. In doing this, you are helping her to make her responses to your verbal cues automatic. But speed up gradually, and do it as a natural outgrowth of *her* progress.

Mastery of these exercises is essential to maintaining stamina during labor. You will be learning specific breathing techniques to cope with each contraction. But controlled relaxation is the means by which energy can be conserved to carry out the techniques in labor. Babies, especially first babies, are not born in an instant. First labors can range from eight to twenty hours, with shorter and longer exceptions of course. Your wife will not work hard this whole time. But if the laboring woman cannot relax to the fullest, the time alone can be exhausting.

As a coach, it is your job to help her to relax during, as well as in between, contractions. To be able to do this, you must master together the controlled relaxation exercises and develop your cue system. In practice sessions, you must be observant, helpful, and patient. It is easy to be critical when you are watching someone else struggle. For the good of these sessions, it would be wise if after you put your wife through the first session, you get down on the floor and let her give you the cues. It is not really as easy as it looks. But doing it yourself will help you to understand what your wife is doing, and it will also help you to know what tension areas to look for.

Controlled relaxation is the key to conserving energy during labor. But the actual tools for dealing with labor contractions are the breathing techniques. By performing a particular pattern of behavior in response to each contraction, a woman is able to cope with the contraction and work with it. Concentrating on executing the pattern of behavior in response to the sensation of the contraction creates a complex mental activity.

The total effect is one of relaxed, deliberate behavior. The woman working with labor is entirely occupied. She must be alert for the signals of the contraction and respond by the breathing technique she has learned. This is a situation where the positive, active behavior has been substituted for a fearful, passive one.

The prepared woman is confident because she is aware of the labor process. She understands the reason why she feels a particular sensation. Her contractions, while they may be uncomfortable to varying degrees, are bearable. She is in control. To be in this position, your wife needs your support and encouragement. Just as with controlled relaxation, you must practice together. Once a day together is sufficient. But it must be every day. Your wife, of course, will be practicing her breathing techniques at least two more sessions each day.

BREATHING TECHNIQUES

The breathing techniques to be used in labor are designed to be natural extensions of normal breathing patterns. The normal patterns have been modified so that a deliberate, conscious effort must be made to carry out the technique as a concentration-response during labor. It is imperative that the breathing be practiced so that in your wife's mind a connection is automatically made between the thought "Contraction begins" and the response "Breathe." During the day when she practices, your wife can say "Contraction begins" to herself and "Contraction ends" when she has finished a breathing technique. But when you practice together, you must give the verbal cues.

Breathing techniques are geared for different levels of labor. In the beginning, there will be no need for control as the contractions are mild enough not to warrant any. By not beginning until necessary, your wife can again conserve mental and physical energy. As labor progresses, your wife will become more serious. When she can no longer talk or laugh during a contraction, it is time to begin using a breathing technique.

Slow rhythmic chest breathing

The first technique consciously uses slow chest breathing. In times of stress, we tend to breathe faster. The purpose of slow rhythmic chest breathing is to provide a concentration-response and to keep the idea of relaxation paramount. The very act of consciously keeping the breathing slow and controlled has a calming effect. The feeling of control will add to your wife's confidence. And the breathing technique will alleviate the major part of your wife's perceived discomfort.

There are basic elements in all of the breathing techniques. As with controlled relaxation, concentration is facilitated by focusing the eyes on a fixed object. To punctuate the beginning and the end of each contraction, a deep breath is taken, so that both you and your wife are aware and in control of each contraction. In practice it is up to you to say "Contraction begins." You will clock the contraction and you will say "Contraction ends" when the time is over. Most practice contractions should be for sixty seconds. In this way, you will be helping your wife to respond to the mental image of "contraction" and to respond for a minute, which is longer than the duration of most contractions. Finally, all breathing techniques utilize chest breathing.

To practice slow rhythmic chest breathing, give your wife her verbal cue. As the "contraction" begins your wife should take a deep breath, in through her nose; and as she exhales through pursed lips, she should be consciously relaxing her body. Practicing for sixty seconds, she should be breathing in through the nose and out through pursed lips, slowly and rhythmically.

You can count for her if she has difficulty maintaining a rhythm, "In . . . two . . . three"; and "Out . . . two . . . three." The important element is rhythm. Slow and deliberate. She will probably get six to nine breaths to a practice minute; most women seem to settle around eight. When you say "Contraction ends" she should then take a deep breath and relax but without the necessity to continue the concentration.

Notice that you will be practicing for sixty seconds. Most contractions throughout labor are less than a minute in duration. But by practicing for a minute, your wife will find it easier to carry on for the lesser duration. Many women report that slow rhythmic chest breathing is a satisfactory technique for them throughout the major part of labor. However, when labor advances and slow chest breathing is no longer a strong enough tool to cope with labor, there is another breathing technique that can be used. It requires somewhat more concentration. Because of the nature of the technique it is called shallow breathing.

Shallow breathing

Shallow breathing is intended to use the air in the upper parts of the lungs. Most people today do not use the full capacity of their lungs under any circumstances. So it is not difficult to use only the upper part, but it requires practice to control the depth of the breathing sequence. The rationale for using this type of breathing is that by not expanding the chest fully during a contraction, there is less change in the intra-abdominal compression caused by the raising and lowering of the diaphragm. Also, as the uterine muscle does become more irritable as labor progresses, it is desirable to allow it to work without the additional physical pressure of the diaphragm.

Because shallow breathing is less deep, one must breathe more quickly to exchange approximately the same amount of oxygen. Also one must inhale and exhale at about the same depth to prevent an imbalance of gases. In the past, women were taught to emphasize the out-breath and in doing so for a prolonged period they tended to blow off more carbon dioxide (the product of respiration) while taking in insufficient amounts of oxygen. The resulting condition, called hyperventilation, is manifested by tingling of hands or feet or a feeling of dizziness. It is easily remedied by rebreathing one's own air either by cupping hands over nose and mouth or by breathing into a small paper bag.

The converse is occasionally seen. Known as hypoventilation, it is manifested by breathlessness and a feeling of anxiety. This, too, is easily remedied. The woman who feels breathless has only to breathe out hard and restart shallow breathing. Neither condition is permanent, nor is it carried on in the prepared woman long enough to do damage to the baby.

In addition, contraction of the uterine muscle momentarily

diminishes the supply of blood to the baby. So that whatever the mother does during a contraction can have little effect on the baby's blood provided she relaxes and breathes normally in between contractions. Physiologists have demonstrated that a relaxed mother has complete restitution of blood gases between contractions. It is, in fact, the unprepared mother hyperventilating continually in a state of panic who has blood gas discrepancies that can travel across the placenta.

Another reason why hyperventilation or hypoventilation rarely cause severe problems in prepared women is that they are conditions that usually occur with shallow breathing. Utilizing only a small percentage of the vital capacity of the lungs leaves a large area of dead space. That is, all of the lung area below the point of shallow breathing is in contact with previously inhaled air. In between contractions, while relaxing, the woman uses all of the lung area she normally would and effects what is for her a reasonable exchange of gases.

The final reason why hyperventilation is not a severe problem for the trained couple is that they know how to recognize and deal with it. As labor coach, you must be alert to the signs. Your wife may report them but be too occupied to remember what they mean. It is a part of your job to recognize the signs and remind her to rebreathe the air she is exhaling or to hold her breath for a few seconds.

Learning technique

To learn the technique for shallow breathing, focus the eyes, take a deep breath to start and then with lips loosely together, inhale and exhale through the nose a little faster than you normally would. Remember, keep it rhythmic; do not rush. Clock it for one minute. Take a deep breath in through the nose and out through pursed lips. Notice that when breathing quickly through the nose, all of the action should be in the upper chest. The abdomen should not move at all, or at least very little. Most people breathe by moving their abdomens in and out. With slow, rhythmic chest breathing, it is a simple matter to transfer the action from the abdomen to the chest. It is easy to fall back to abdominal breathing when the movement is not on such a large scale. But the essence of shallow breathing is that it is shallow *chest* breathing.

As a coach in the practice sessions, you can help your wife tremendously if she is having trouble keeping her breathing high in the chest. Try one practice contraction by having her place her hands on her abdomen and letting her feel what she is doing. Try the next one by placing your hand lightly on her chest just below her throat and tell her to breathe at your hand. This is a good way to give direction to her breathing.

Once she gets the knack of high chest breathing, the next step in learning shallow breathing is to transfer from nasal breathing to breathing through the mouth. This is to add another focus for concentration as most of us breathe normally through our noses. The transfer is accomplished by allowing the jaw to drop enough to permit the lips to part slightly.

Counteracting dryness

As mouth breathing can be very drying, there are two things to be added here that will counteract dryness as much as is possible. First, a slight smile helps; not a fool's grin. Just enough to bring the corners of the mouth up somewhat. Second, place the tip of the tongue behind the upper front teeth. This helps to direct the current of air under and around the tongue rather than straight across the top. Again, when practicing, Coach, do not forget to check for focused eyes and deep breath at the beginning and end of the contraction, and to supply your verbal cues.

In actual labor, it will be the intensity of the contraction that will guide the rhythm of the shallow breathing. Do not move ahead until your wife can shallow breathe at an even rate, effortlessly for a full minute. In fact, you both should do this as many couples have found it invaluable for the coach to breathe with his wife in labor to help her with the rhythm.

During a contraction, either practice or real, you can make it easier for your wife if you call off the seconds in intervals of ten or fifteen seconds. If this sounds like nonsense to you, try to shallow breathe for one minute with her timing you. Then try another minute with her calling off the seconds. The value of your presence just in calling off seconds becomes patently clear.

Tactile stimulation

To prepare yourselves for coping with actual contractions, you can practice responding to tactile stimulation. The contractions in labor will be best perceived by your wife. She will *feel* the beginning of the muscular tension long before someone outside her body can monitor the tightening in her abdomen. That interval can best be used to gather her resources, focus her eyes, and take the deep breath that signals that the contraction has begun.

In labor, you will be working together to cope with the contraction as it builds to its peak and then subsides. You can help your wife get ready for this. What you must do is provide a substitute for a contraction. This is excellent practice for her to learn how to respond to what she actually perceives. It involves the same kind of concentration as she will need to use to work along with the rhythm of labor.

To practice, rest your hand on your wife's upper arm or thigh. She is to begin her breathing technique as you increase pressure by slowly squeezing her limb. You should increase the pressure as a contraction would build: beginning slowly, building to a peak in about fifteen seconds, holding the peak for about twenty seconds, and gradually declining, making a total of between forty-five and fifty seconds. Your wife's response should be to focus her eyes and take a deep breath as the pressure begins. To begin, she should use moderate shallow breathing, increasing the tempo with the pressure she feels and decreasing the tempo as she feels the pressure decrease. As with all contractions, she should end with a deep breath.

You will find that with practice, your wife will be able to respond automatically to this practice technique. It requires intense mental effort to concentrate on the physical sensation and respond to it with a learned breathing technique. In addition, it will give your wife practice at excluding distractions. Extraneous sounds or movement in her peripheral vision must not be allowed to interfere with her effort to concentrate.

Concentrating

We all have been in situations where we are said to be absorbed in a book or a movie. All of our attention is given to that activity to the temporary exclusion of all other sensory stimuli. So it must be in labor. You can help your wife to sharpen her ability to concentrate. Without prior discussion, hum a few bars of a song during a practice contraction; adjust her collar; move your hand just outside her line of sight. To the average person, any one of these distractions would be attention catching. But the prepared woman must make special effort to keep her eyes focused on a fixed point and her mind focused on the contraction-breathing relationship going on in her body.

You can help her in labor by running interference. Should someone speak to her or ask a question during a contraction, you should speak up. Politely remind that person that your wife is concentrating and you are sure that she would be happy to talk to them after the contraction has ended. If you can accurately answer for her, you might do that. Although you will probably find that your answer would be verified by your wife anyway, do not fall in the habit of always speaking for her. True you are working together. However, she is the one who is in labor. She alone feels the sensations. She may have something to say about the quality of her labor that you from the outside cannot perceive. Therefore, if she is able, let her speak for herself. If she is occupied, then you speak for her, if you can.

Adding effleurage

Up to this point the discussion has been focused largely on the breathing techniques. There is another component of behavior that is used in conjunction with the breathing when a stronger tool is needed. Called effleurage from the French meaning "light touch," this pattern of delicate stroking is added to the breathing patterns when more concentration is required to maintain control. Also by providing a featherlike massage to the abdominal muscles, effleurage is comforting to many women.

The practice of effleurage is always in conjunction with a breathing technique. It can be done with slow rhythmic chest breathing, and it can be done with shallow breathing either in its continued rhythm form or in its accelerated and decelerated form. The basic effleurage technique involves selective relaxation. Arms and shoulders are relaxed except for those muscles necessary to move them. Starting position is loose wrists, fingertips barely touching the skin on the lower abdomen just above the pubic hair.

With slow chest breathing, the effleurage accompanies the breathing as follows: with the deep breath at the beginning, the hands assume starting position. With each inhalation, the hands move around and up the outside of the abdomen meeting at the top. With the exhalation, the fingertips move straight down the abdomen, passing the umbilicus (navel) to return to the starting position to begin the circle again with the next inhalation.

With shallow breathing, special effort must be made to keep the effleurage slow and light. The tendency is to become frantic. Not only would this rapidly lead to fatigue, it would cause unnecessary anxiety and, probably, irritation to the skin of the abdomen. To remain calm, practice effleurage with the shallow breathing as follows: while taking a deep breath at the beginning, bring hands to starting position. Begin the effluerage with the first shallow breath.

The pattern of the effleurage is coordinated with the breathing pattern. With the first four breaths, the hands rise halfway around the arc of the abdomen. With the next four breaths, the hands reach the top of the abdomen. With the third series of four breaths, the hands come halfway down the abdomen, about the level of the umbilicus. With the next four breaths, the hands come back to the starting position ready to begin again. It does require quite a bit of effort to match the effleurage to breathing, as well as to remain relaxed and keep the touch light.

Using the effleurage with the accelerated shallow breathing utilizes the same pattern. The only difference is that as the breathing accelerates, the effleurage accelerates to keep pace, and it decelerates as the breathing does. Special effort must be made to keep arms relaxed as there is a strong tendency to become tense with acceleration.

As a coach, you should be watching to see that your wife is relaxed. Observe her head, neck, shoulders, and hands. Even though she is moving her arms, there is no reason for her shoulders to be hunched up or tense; this is a common reaction when effluerage is first added to the breathing. Remind her to relax.

Effluerage is an adjunct to breathing. It is not an essential part which must be included. Some women find that they dislike the sensation of a light touch. Some women find that they concentrate better in actual labor without the effleurage. Still others find that in labor effleurage tires them, and they ask their husbands to do the effleurage for them. Unless you plan to go through labor with your wife sitting in your lap, it is obvious that you could not do the effleurage as described above.

When the husband does the effleurage, movement is modified so that he is lightly touching the areas of discomfort. These areas are the circle created by the wall of the uterus inside the abdominal wall and the part of the lower abdomen over the expanding cervix. Starting position for the husband, therefore, is to place the fingers of one hand lightly on the upper part of his wife's abdomen on the side away from him. He then can slowly bring his hand down the outer part of his wife's abdomen, across the lower abdomen and along the outer side of the abdomen on the side close to him. You would begin again by lifting your hand and returning to starting position.

To keep the light touch from becoming uncomfortable as a result of friction to the skin, it is wise to use fine talcum powder. Baby powder is the best as strong floral scents may distress your wife in labor. Besides, you will be able to find a use for any that is left over.

Technique for transition

The final breathing technique for labor is designed to give your wife control during the shortest and most difficult period. Named transition, this period occurs just before the baby makes his final descent to be born. At this point, the cervix, the opening through which the baby must pass, has not quite yet expanded to its fullest diameter. Instead of being ten centimeters, it may be only eight centimeters.

You can see from the number that most of the work of labor is over. But, at this point, although the baby's head is causing internal pressure which will give your wife the urge to push, it is too soon. It will take only a few contractions more until the cervix is fully dilated. If however, your wife pushes before full dilatation, the additional pressure on the cervix can cause edema, or swelling, which can prolong this particularly uncomfortable phase of labor.

Your doctor will examine her frequently and give permission to push as soon as he feels there is full dilatation. Until then, it will be necessary for your wife to work at trying not to push. For this she needs to know the pant-blow breathing technique.

The rationale for this technique is that blowing out in short, staccato breaths counters the urge to push. But since the urge to push is not constant and the contraction itself is difficult to control, a strong pattern of breathing is necessary. The combination designed to meet both of these requirements is the pant-blow rhythm. It is used in the following way: a deep breath is taken quickly because the contraction builds very rapidly. Then a pattern of six shallow pants and one, short, staccato blow is begun immediately.

Countering urge to push

This pattern is maintained until the urge to push becomes strong. To counter the urge to push, the woman should blow-blow-blow continually until it passes, returning to the pant-blow rhythm. This should be repeated as many times as necessary during a contraction. End the contraction with a deep breath. Since relaxation is so difficult during transition contractions, it is a good idea to encourage your wife to consciously relax and do rhythmic chest breathing in between them.

It is the nature of the contraction during transition that makes this phase so difficult. Up until this point, contractions build to a peak and decline. In transition, they may build very quickly, peak, partially decline, and peak again. It is this erratic characteristic that makes them so hard to control. Add to this the extremely short rest intervals in between contractions and you can understand why your wife will need so much help at this time in her labor.

Coaching during transition requires firmness, as well as encouragement. Your wife will be very tired. It would not be unusual if her big muscles trembled. Nor is it uncommon for women in transition to be nauseated or even vomit. You can expect your wife to be irritable, argumentative, and even abusive. This is the time she needs your firm support most.

In transition, most women cannot think too clearly. Contract-tions are very strong and require all of their attention. Tell your wife what she has to do. Help her to begin at the beginning of the contraction. Keep reminding her that she is doing a great job and that the baby is almost here. *Never* leave your wife during a contraction. In between contractions, go find the doctor and ask him to examine your wife to know if she may have permission to push. Be sure you tell her before you go that you are going to get the doctor. He will be nearby.

When your wife is given permission to push, you will see a most dramatic change in her. Pushing is the final lap, and she can almost see the finish line. The contractions when she can push become more manageable again. And being able to push is such a tremendous relief that she will suddenly find renewed energy. Finally, pushing marks the end of labor and the beginning of delivery.

Pushing effectively, just as coping with labor, requires practice. Of course, babies are born every day of mothers who are fully anesthetized and therefore in no condition to consciously push. But by learning to push properly, your wife can substantially reduce the time of the expulsive stage. This means that the baby will be born in a shorter time. For him this means less pressure on his body from the forces of birth. For your wife it means less pressure on her internal organs, which means that she is lessening the chances of developing "female" problems later in life.

Limiting pushing practice

In practicing pushing, it is necessary to understand the position and process without actually executing the maneuver as it would be in labor. The reason for this is that many obstetricians feel that continued hard pushing against a closed cervix is not the same either physically or perceptually and if the woman has problems that occur in the course of pregnancy, such as hemorrhoids, straining to push against the closed cervix may well aggravate them. So, although the position is assumed and the breathing is done, the actual pushing effort in practice is limited to no more than ten or fifteen seconds.

A preliminary exercise will be of enormous help in getting your wife's body ready for pushing. Your wife has been doing the Kegel, or perineal tightening, exercise since she began her physical fitness for pregnancy program. She should have pretty good control of contracting and releasing those muscles. The next step, which is the preliminary exercise for pushing, is to selectively contract those muscles in a progression and relax in the opposite progression.

As a man, you just do not have the equipment to do this. But you can understand the exercise by thinking of an elevator at the street level. Then imagine that the elevator rises: first floor . . . second floor . . . third floor . . . hold it . . . hold it. Going down: second floor . . . first floor . . . street floor . . . basement. Push out.

It is the last step, pushing out at the basement floor, that will help your wife to understand and feel the direction and nature of the pushing.

Position for pushing

Most primiparas (women pregnant with their first babies) push initially in the labor room. They are only too willing to begin pushing the moment they are given permission by the doctor. Your job as coach will be to see that your wife is in a good position to push. She should be resting supine on two pillows arranged so that one is doubled under her shoulders and the other is lying the long way so that it extends down her back. This will give her a wedge of just the right height for effective pushing. Any higher, the tendency is for the woman to raise herself almost to a sitting position when she is pushing. The angle then of her pelvis serves as a deterrent to her efforts.

As the contraction begins, your wife should breathe in, out, in, out, in, and hold it. This pattern allows the contraction to

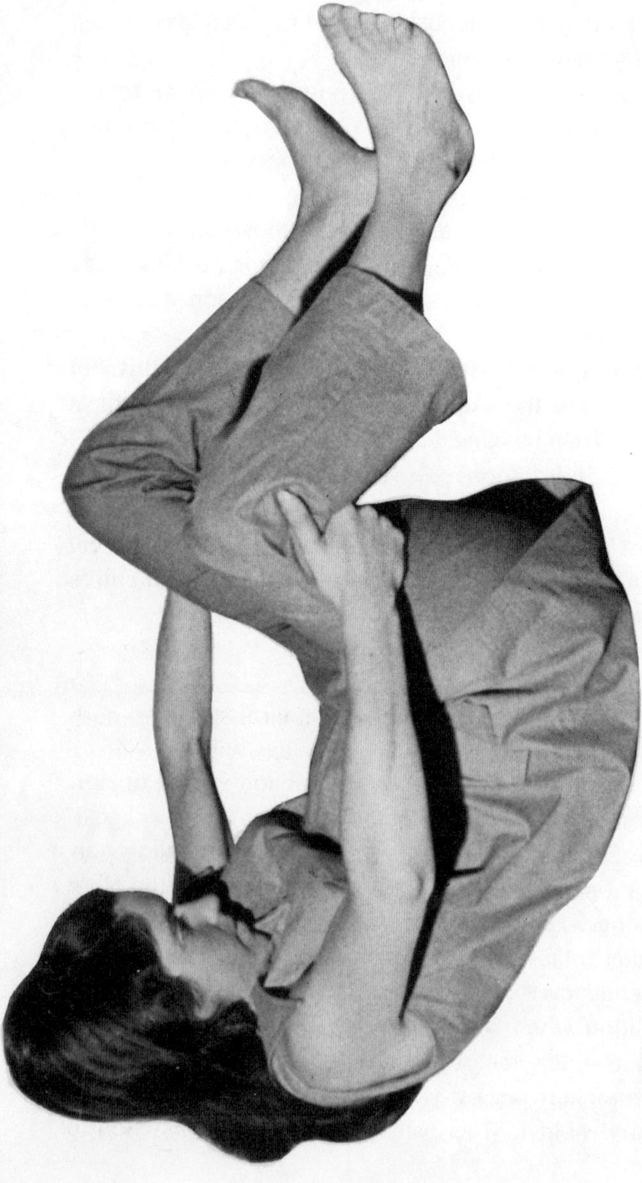

Figure 14. *POSITION FOR PUSHING: Points to check—are shoulders round? is head down? are elbows out? are feet relaxed?*

reach its peak so that she will be pushing with it when it is strongest. As she holds her breath by blocking the air in her lungs, she should round her shoulders, grasp her knees keeping her elbows out, consciously relax her perineum, and push. You can help by supporting one or both of her legs. As she feels she needs more air, she can turn her head, let the air explode out of her lungs, and immediately take another breath.

All this is done quickly while she continues to maintain the downward pushing of the thoracic and abdominal muscles. In labor you can remind your wife to keep her lips relaxed. If her mouth is tight, it is a good clue to you that her perineum is tense also. Be sure you check all points: round shoulders, elbows out, lips relaxed. Keep telling her what a good job she is doing.

In labor, you and your wife will have to decide how she is most comfortable for pushing. Some women prefer the position described. Others find that the weight of their legs is too much for them to support, and they ask their husbands to support the legs during pushing efforts. Others find that they prefer to have their husbands support their shoulders. And many women who have long legs find that they are most comfortable if they grasp their ankles. The elbows are not out in this position because the arms pass under the legs to reach the ankles. But the legs are in just as good a position as they are well supported and wide apart to allow the baby maximum room for moving down. Since the reason for having elbows out is to encourage the women to get their knees far apart for effective pushing, the latter position is of help to an overly modest woman who can not otherwise assume the proper position.

If you are supporting your wife's legs, you will be in an ideal position for watching her perineum. As the baby's head moves down, you will be able to see the perineum bulge out toward you a little. Gradually you will be able to see small patches of the top of the baby's head peak out at you while she pushes. Tell her! Share your excitement. She needs to know and will work even harder knowing that the baby is practically here. When you can see a patch about the size of a quarter, the doctor will take you and your wife down to the delivery room.

Pushing in the delivery room is the same as pushing in the labor room except your wife's legs will be supported in stirrups. You can practice for this by using a straight back chair. Your wife should lie on the floor with her buttocks touching the legs of the chair and her legs resting on the seat. Since your place in the delivery room will be at your wife's head, practice coaching her from that spot. Become familiar with the way the proper position should look from your vantage point. Practice from directly behind her head and from a point off each shoulder. In that way, you will know what to look for from any angle you might encounter.

This chapter is not intended to be a full or complete training guide. It is intended to present the philosophy and techniques of psychoprophylaxis training from the father's point of view. Couples cannot be urged strongly enough to attend the classes given by accredited childbirth educators.

Points about training

1) Practice every day until delivery. Your wife should have three practice sessions during the day, one of which is a session with you as her coach.

2) Controlled relaxation is the key to preventing fatigue. Perfect the ability to selectively relax muscle groups. Practice sitting, reclining, side-lying.

3) Breathing techniques are tools for coping with contractions. There are basic elements to all breathing techniques used in PPM: a) deep breathe beginning and end of contraction; b) focus eyes; c) think "chest;" d) relax all muscle groups not actively working; e) the contraction-rhythm-intensity determines the breathing response; and f) effleurage, if added control is needed (optional).

3

Going to the Hospital

As part of your childbirth education course, you will learn what to expect when you and your wife finally go the hospital. That is the time when your having attended classes will pay off. You will be prepared and ready to act as labor coach, a role you have been practicing at home.

Late in the eighth or early in the ninth month of your wife's pregnancy, you and your wife should take a tour of the hospital where your baby will be delivered. This timing will allow for your memory to still be fresh when your wife's labor begins, and it allows you enough of a margin to be able to make the tour even if your baby arrives early.

Your hospital may have a regularly scheduled tour for expectant parents. By contacting the maternity supervisor, you can set up a date to attend the tour. If the hospital does not have a regular tour, the maternity supervisor can arrange one especially for you. Of course you will make the request in your most gentlemanly manner. You gain a lot more by politely asking for help than by demanding your rights.

While you are making the tour, you should notice particularly where you are supposed to wait while your wife is going through admissions procedure. Some hospitals provide a special area for fathers to wait. Others expect you to be in the lobby. Still others will want you to be near the nurses' station right on the labor floor so that you can be assisted into a hospital gown, over your street clothes, and escorted into the labor room at the first possible moment.

The tour date would probably be the best time for you to plan your route and to make a test run. Time the distance from your house to the hospital. Decide which route will be quickest and most direct. This is the time to plan possible alternate routes, especially if you live in a metropolitan area in which traffic becomes particularly congested during the morning and evening rush hours. Near the hospital, locate a place where you can leave your car for an undetermined period. If you are travelling by public transportation, be sure to locate the proper transfer points and note the distances to be walked at each end.

RECOGNIZING AND PREPARING FOR LABOR

When you have settled the mechanics of getting to the hospital, you are ready to turn your attention to recognizing and preparing for the onset of labor.

As the time draws near for the baby to be born, you and your wife will grow more and more restless with anticipation. Every time the baby moves, she will wait anxiously for contractions to begin. Every time you see her belly tighten, as it does quite normally during the latter part of pregnancy, you will be ready to pull out your stopwatch and begin timing. This will seem the longest month of your lives.

There is only one word of caution. Birth is a normal event. You have hired the services of a highly competent obstetrician. You have prepared yourselves so that when labor begins you will both be ready to participate in this childbirth experience. Do not, repeat, do not take yourselves so seriously that you lose all perspective. Labor will take place whether or not you participate.

You chose to participate so that you could provide physical and emotional assistance to your wife. Psychoprophylaxis is a relatively comfortable way of having a baby with dignity. It requires the cooperative efforts of a team—your wife, yourself, your obstetrician, the childbirth educator, and the hospital staff. This is not a crusade, nor is it a contest. Nobody gets any medals for martyrdom. Maintain your perspective and remain within your role as labor coach.

Labor is a unique experience for each woman. The exact length, the number of contractions, the duration of any phase of labor vary from woman to woman and from labor to labor in the same woman. But the majority of women follow a very predictable pattern. With most first babies, labor can last from twelve to twenty hours. This includes all of the time from the first barely perceptible contraction to the moment when the cervix is completely dilated and the baby is ready to make his final descent and be born.

Contractions of labor are the involuntary shortening and tightening of the uterine muscles for the purpose of expanding or dilating the cervix so that the baby can get from inside to outside your wife. In the last few months of pregnancy, you and your wife may have noticed that periodically her abdomen seems to get very tight and then relax. It is not a particularly uncomfortable sensation, though it may be disconcerting if you do not understand what you are seeing.

Braxton-Hicks contractions

What you have seen and she has felt are contractions. They are called Braxton-Hicks contractions or sometimes false labor. These contractions are not really labor, but they are doing the job of preparing the uterus and the cervix for labor to begin. They can be distinguished from true labor by the way they occur. Braxton-Hicks contractions usually do not establish a pattern that indicates progress. That is, while they may occur at intervals of ten minutes for several hours, they never get any closer or any stronger. But they do have a job to do. They work silently. Some women are not even aware these mild contractions are occurring.

The reason that all the fuss is made about Braxton-Hicks contractions is that in their great desire to have labor finally begin, many couples mistakenly identify the beginning of labor with Braxton-Hicks contractions. This is not a big crime. But it may necessitate an unnecessary trip to the doctor which can be very disappointing to the woman who wants so much for her labor to start.

Show; ruptured membranes

Whether or not labor is really established can only be determined by your obstetrician's making an internal examination of the cervix. However, there are a number of signs which will give you a pretty good idea that this is it. First, as the cervix effaces, or thins down, a mucous plug which has guarded the baby from the outside world can no longer be contained by the changing cervix and is expelled.

Remember, when labor begins, the cervix is long and narrow and its walls are quite thick, somewhat like a tunnel. When the mucous plug separates from the inside of the tunnel, small capillaries give way and the mucous is mixed with tiny amounts of blood which makes it pinkish. This blood-tinged mucous is called show. It is eliminated from the body through the vagina. If your wife has not yet been aware of contractions, this painless discharge may come as a pleasant surprise. You can expect contractions to begin, or that is, for her to become aware of them shortly.

Another sign that would indicate that labor is underway is the rupture of membranes. That sounds horrendously painful, does it not? Well, it is not. The membrane, or amniotic sac, is a thin covering surrounding the baby and the amniotic fluid which has served as a bumper against collisions from the outside world. There are no nerve endings in the membrane. So neither mother nor baby can actually feel them.

As labor progresses and the cervix begins to dilate, a portion of the membrane protrudes through the opening. The succeeding contractions continue to apply pressure to this portion of the membrane. It is similar to trying to force a balloon full of water through a narrow hole. The pressure from the contractions increases the internal pressure from the fluid causing the portion of the membrane protruding through the opening to expand until it reaches its limit. Then it pops. When this happens, your wife will probably experience a sudden gush or a steady trickle of liquid. At any rate, this tells you that the cervix has begun to dilate.

It is a good idea to place a rubber sheet under your bottom sheet during the last month of pregnancy. Then if your wife's membranes rupture during the night, she has not soaked a good mattress.

Finally, the nature of the contractions themselves are an indication that true labor has begun. Braxton-Hicks contractions are often felt as tightening in the front of the abdomen. True labor often, though not always, begins as a recurrent low backache which radiates around to the front. As the contractions continue over a period of time, they last longer, feel stronger, and occur closer together. This is what is meant when labor is said to be progressive.

A good way to see if the contractions are actual labor or not is to have your wife get up and walk around. Braxton-Hicks will usually subside with activity; true labor will not. This is a good time for your wife to take a shower and wash her hair. It serves two purposes. First, it will be a few days before she can wash her hair if this is true labor. And, second, if she is still contracting after that maneuver, it probably is.

If you and your wife find cocktails relaxing, the onset of labor is an ideal time to make yourselves a favorite drink. Starting out relaxed is the key to a happy experience. After you leisurely finish your cocktail, it will be time to get down to the business of observing and taking over your job as labor coach.

THE ONSET OF LABOR

Initially, you should time a series of contractions and note any other signs of labor that occur and report these to your obstetrician. If your call is close to his office hours, he may suggest you bring your wife in so he can confirm her progress. At any rate he will probably want to talk to your wife to confirm your report. If he feels that it is really early labor and you are both in control, he may be satisfied to tell you to keep in contact by telephone, reporting your wife's progress or any changes.

Many obstetricians who regularly practice psychoprophylaxis have come to trust the accuracy of reporting and the judgment of trained couples. They also recognize the advisability of delaying admission to the hospital until it is time for the obstetrical team to function together.

Most labors, especially with first babies, have a fairly long period of mild to moderate contractions. This is the time when the woman is usually in complete control without any need for breathing techniques. She may find that walking is more comfortable than sitting or lying down. She can be easily distracted by some activity such as knitting, reading, or watching television. The last point has led some people to refer to this as the entertainment phase. Since hospitals are not designed to provide for such activities and usually confine the laboring woman to bed, it makes good sense to be in the calm atmosphere of home where such activities are readily available for this period of time.

In the early part of labor, you need to encourage your wife to be involved in other things as long as she is comfortable. Too often, the woman focuses her whole attention on the contractions at the time she should be able to do other things. In absorbing herself with the contractions, her perception of them becomes distorted. Because she wants so very much to have labor move along, she perceives the contractions as stronger than they are. This honest belief leads her to begin breathing techniques when they are not yet necessary.

Your job as coach

As labor coach, your job is to help her get involved in a quiet activity. Your goals are: 1) to keep her mind occupied so that the perception of the early contractions does not get out of proportion, 2) to help her to rest as much as possible to conserve her energy for the work she is to do later, and 3) to be available so that your wife feels that someone she loves is nearby and competent to help her. Your mood should be cheerful. After all, labor has started.

If you can both sleep during this period of early labor, you will be doing yourselves a favor to do so. However, if it is the time of day you are normally wide awake, watch a television program or go to a movie. Be sure to tell your obstetrician your whereabouts. And, for goodness sake, pick a light movie. This is no time for deep soul-searching messages. Nor is it a time for dramatic tales of parent-child conflicts. The purpose of going to a movie is to relax and permit the early part of labor to happen without undue attention. You may find that you never finish the story. As labor progresses, your wife will no longer be content to sit through each contraction doing nothing. She may wish to walk. Or she may be ready to begin using a breathing technique.

Your prime function as labor coach at this time is to see that you and your wife get as much rest as possible. You will both need as much energy and stamina as you are able to conserve when the working part of labor begins in earnest.

You will also be recording the progress of labor for the doctor. However, it is not necessary to sit up all night to watch each contraction. He will be most interested in knowing how labor has changed over a period of time. So, you can time a series of contractions—five or six—and go back to sleep, if possible and then when you wake up begin timing again. The obstetrician will be interested in knowing how frequently the contractions occur and how long they last. You will note by the clock the time each contraction begins. The beginning of one contraction to the beginning of the next is the interval that is measured to express the frequency of contractions.

Measuring duration

To measure the duration, if your wife is using a breathing technique, you can note the number of seconds from the time she took her deep breath to begin her breathing exercise until she takes her deep breath that signals the end. You can also time the duration of a contraction by lightly placing your hand on the fundus which is the large rounded part of the uterus at the top of the abdomen. This will tighten and become hard to the touch as the muscles contract and become soft again as they relax between contractions. As this requires some practice you may wish to time the breathing and feel the contraction at the same time until you can recognize either equally well.

You might even try to time Braxton-Hicks contractions by touch, if your wife has a series of them. Remember, however, to keep your touch light. A heavy touch can cause unnecessary muscular irritability. The pressure of your hand should be just enough for you to feel the muscles change condition. Men sometimes forget just how heavy their own well-muscled hands are.

In addition to noting the characteristics of the contractions per se, you should also note your wife's mood or anything that you think is unusual. Your comments along these lines will help the doctor in appraising the progress of labor.

Consider the following sample as a possible form for your notes:

SAMPLE LABOR DIARY

Contraction begins	Duration	Technique	Comments
6:00 AM	30 secs	none	At last it's started — bloody show present — Mary excited — no discomfort, except backache
6:20 AM	35 secs	none	
6:50 AM	40 secs	none	
7:00 AM	30 secs	none	
7:10 AM	40 secs	none	
7:20 AM	40 secs	none	
7:30 AM	45 secs	none	Called doctor
10:00 AM	50 secs	slow chest	Mary busy during contraction — still talking, joking between — seems comfortable — using slow chest
10:07 AM	45 secs	slow chest	
10:17 AM	45 secs	slow chest	
10:25 AM	50 secs	slow chest	
10:35 AM	45 secs	slow chest	Mary wet — no discomfort small amounts of fluid, not urine — called doctor

Before leaving home

While you are still at home, remind your wife to urinate. She may not feel the urge although her bladder may be at least partially full. Assist her to the bathroom in between contractions. Stay nearby so that if a contraction does begin, she does not feel left alone with it. Emptying the bladder is important throughout labor as a full bladder by itself can act as a mechanical retardant to the progress of labor.

By the time she is doing any breathing technique your wife should not be eating. Check with your obstetrician; he may permit his patients to eat lightly. But most physicians limit their patients in early labor to clear liquids—jello or tea with sugar. This permits them to keep up their fluids and get a little energy from the carbohydrates. But the ability of the stomach to digest slows almost to a standstill during labor.

Fats and proteins eaten in early labor often remain in the stomach, undigested, for hours. This can lead to exaggerated nausea and unpleasant vomiting late in labor or at delivery. And vomiting can be a danger to your wife as the consequences of aspirating vomitus into the lungs can be fatal.

But do not let your wife's limitation on food affect you. You should eat. Food may be hard to come by without leaving your wife once she is in the hospital. Some men bring along a sandwich for the time in the labor room and one for their wives to eat after delivery.

Although most women have their bags packed well in advance of their due date, it might be well to match the contents against a checklist to see that you both have everything that you need.

For the trained couple two bags should be packed. One is the traditional suitcase which has all the toilet articles and bedclothes needed for a three to four day stay in the hospital.

The second bag is for the labor room, and you should carry it. The suitcase will most probably be removed from the labor area and taken to the room your wife will occupy on the postpartum floor. So anything you want to keep with you should be in the labor room bag. You will need your tools to help your wife:

1) Powder—to minimize friction on the skin during effluerage or backrubs. Choose a powder that smells fresh such as a baby powder as an overly perfumed powder tends to nauseate a woman in advanced labor.

2) Chapstick—a lip balm helps to keep your wife's lips moist while she is doing the breathing techniques.

WHAT TO TAKE TO THE HOSPITAL

SUITCASE	*LABOR ROOM BAG*
two nightgowns, washable	powder
one robe, washable	chapstick
one pair slippers	mouthwash
brush and comb	two clean tennis balls
toothbrush and toothpaste	two cans of frozen fruit juice
soap (if preference)	variety of tart lollipops
shampoo	a picture
two maternity bras	two sandwiches
one sanitary belt (as spare)	paper bag, sandwich size
make-up (optional)	

3) *Mouthwash*—most people have a preference for a mouthwash flavor and while the hospital can usually supply something, it may not be to your wife's liking. As she is not likely to take much by mouth, the mouthwash will probably be important to her and should be a flavor she likes.

4) *Tennis balls*—if back pressure becomes a real problem, counterpressure is usually the most effective answer. Two clean tennis balls are ideal when placed between your wife's aching back and the bed. It will give you a respite, leaving you free to do other things for her (see section on back labor for details).

5) *Cans of frozen juice*—these can be a means of providing cold and pressure. But any application of heat or cold should only be with the permission of the physician.

6) *Lollipops*—preferably sour flavors as the others cloy. Any candy to be used in labor must have a stick so that you can remove it from your wife's mouth when a contraction begins if she does not think to do it. This is to prevent any accidents resulting from whole swallowed candies.

7) *A picture*—it is nice to have a favorite picture to focus the eyes on during a contraction. Be sure to bring masking tape to hang it as tacks and cellophane tape mar the hospital walls.

8) *Two sandwiches*—one for you, in case you get hungry during labor; one for your wife after she delivers. For while you will be in a hospital with facilities to serve several hundreds of people, it may not be serving time when you become hungry or after your wife delivers.

9) *Paper bag*—this bag should be the size for sandwiches so that it can be used for your wife to rebreathe exhaled air if she feels dizzy. If the bag is much larger, it becomes unwieldy and defeats its purpose.

Just as there are things you will want to take to the hospital, there are things you should leave home. Jewelry is the prime example. You should make sure that your wife leaves all her jewelry home, with the possible exception of her wedding ring. She will only be asked to remove it and give it to you at the hospital. So, why risk losing it?

You *will* need the watch you have been using for practice sessions. Although most labor rooms have large, visible wall clocks, you will probably be most comfortable with your own watch.

Your obstetrician will tell you when he wants your wife to be brought to the hospital. But it is your responsibility to keep him informed. He will let you know whether he will call you at regular intervals or whether he wants you to call him. Either way have your record sheet handy to the telephone. Have the essential information summarized in your mind: "My wife's contractions are so many minutes apart, lasting so many seconds. She ruptured her membranes at such and such o'clock. She is doing slow chest breathing with no effleurage. She seems comfortable and in control."

ADMISSION PROCEDURES

When you do bring your wife to the hospital, you can expect an interval of anywhere from one-half an hour to an hour when you will be separated. This time is devoted to the admission procedures.

If you have not already provided the necessary information by preregistration, you will be asked to register your wife and indicate the method of payment you will be making at the admissions office. Therefore to avoid any unnecessary unpleasantness and delay, remember to bring along any forms or policy holder cards you might need to verify your membership in your hospitalization plan. Any other arrangements can be clarified at that time also.

Meanwhile, your wife will have been whisked away to the labor floor. Admissions procedure for her means a whole routine of identification and preparation for any eventuality.

First, a doctor, probably a resident physician if your hospital is a teaching hospital, will examine your wife. He will do an internal examination to determine at what point in labor your wife actually is. This information will be relayed to your own obstetrician. Then a nurse will check her temperature, pulse, and blood pressure. Your wife will be asked for a urine specimen.

A blood sample will be taken at this time so that in the rare event that there is an emergency, blood which your wife's body can accept will be available. There is no cost to you for blood that is not used, and the investment in the blood test is well worth the expense in case there is need for the blood later. Finally, your wife will be given an enema and the skin around the delivery area will be prepared, or shaved, so that it is as clean as possible.

These last two items have drawn the most attention of the entire admissions procedure. Obstetricians vary in the emphasis they place on the importance of them. But if your obstetrician endorses these two steps, you should understand why they have survived other changes in obstetrical care.

Bascially, the enema is given for two reasons. First, it empties the bowels. As most women are constipated at the end of pregnancy, this cleaning out is helpful to provide maximum room for labor to take place. Also, if a woman knows her lower bowel is empty, she can push much more effectively without being afraid that she will have an accident and embarrass herself. Second, the enema itself provides mechanical stimulation to the uterus. The tempo of labor will pick up after the enema.

Some women have arrived at the hospital having already given themselves an enema. This may or may not be accepted as sufficient. If you and your wife have any such plans, check it out with your physician first. At best an enema is uncomfortable. It would be a shame to put your wife through it twice unnecessarily.

The same kinds of remarks can be made about the prep, or the shaving of the perineal area. Preps are now done in a variety of ways. Some doctors still feel that to ensure the baby's well-being, all pubic, vulval, and perineal hair should be removed and the skin painted with an antiseptic solution. Hair, they believe, is a breeding ground for bacteria and must be removed to prevent the spread of infection. Other equally competent obstetricians are satisfied that a modified prep, which involves only the vulval and perineal hair, is sufficient.

Yes, it is true that the hair growing back itches and is prickly for a short while. If it is a big thing for your wife, have her talk to your obstetrician. But do not waste your time playing barber on the way to the hospital. No matter how careful you are, it just is not like shaving your own face. Not only will the shave be questionable and probably repeated, but there is a pretty good chance that small nicks in the sensitive skin will become infected.

By the time your wife's routine is completed, you should be finished with your business at the admissions office.

When you enter the labor room, do not be surprised if the calm, slow breathing wife you left at the admissions office looks a little panicky. It is really amazing how the presence of a competent husband can get her back on the track. Keep *your* cool. Greet her warmly. Start doing your job just as you were doing it at home. It is very comforting to the woman in labor to have familiar things going on, such as your timing her contractions and your reminding her to relax tense areas.

THE LABOR ROOM

In between contractions, set up the labor room for your convenience. Put the supplies you brought in your labor room bag within easy reach. If you want to sit, pull up a chair so that you are near your wife. You will want to be near enough to touch her during contractions—to check for relaxation or to do the effleurage for her if she asks you. Confer with her about where she wants her picture hung so she can focus on it most easily.

Find out if your wife is in a comfortable position. Too often, women in labor are left flat in bed, largely because they are heavily sedated and are not aware of their own comfort or discomfort. But just as it is uncomfortable late in pregnancy to be flat, so it is during labor. And yet, most women are so bewildered by the admissions procedure that they do not think clearly enough to change position even if they are uncomfortable. Labor will continue if she stands on her head. So find out how she will be most relaxed.

Familiarize yourself with the hospital bed. Most of these beds are mechanical, with two cranks operated by arm-power. One crank located at one corner of the foot of the bed controls the head of the bed—it can be raised or lowered depending on which way the crank is rotated. The other crank controls the foot of the bed—raising or lowering it about knee level. Its use is not usually recommended, however, because when the lower half of the bed is cranked it tends to put pressure on the blood vessels located in the back of the woman's legs. It is better to position the legs with pillows if they are available.

Changing the bed is only one way you can assist your wife to change position. You can help her to sit tailor fashion. Women who experienced back pressure in labor find this an effective change. To accomplish this position in bed, raise the head of the bed to its highest point and place her pillows behind her back and head so that she can relax fully in this sitting position. Whatever her position, your goal is to see that your wife does not have to support any part of her body unnecessarily, such as her head or her arms. This conserves her energy.

Another position many women find comfortable in labor is side-lying. You can assist your wife to side-lie. This puts the weight of the baby on the bed. And it also gives you access to her back if she would find it comforting to have you rub it. For side-lying you would lower the bed to its flat position. When your wife has turned on her side, place one pillow under her top leg so it is supported and one pillow under her top arm. In this position, with her limbs supported, she can rest without straining either hip or shoulder.

These are not the only positions. Experiment with whatever variations of sitting or lying she finds comfortable. Most hospitals do not allow the woman in labor out of bed. This is intended to prevent accidents. Find out your hospital's policy and your doctor's feelings about this before you even attempt such a maneuver.

If you *know* you have permission, your wife may be most comfortable sitting in a stuffed chair that is usually in most labor rooms. Or she may find that walking is most helpful. If so, you should be at her side with one arm around her waist and the other supporting her elbow nearest you. She definitely *should not* be out of bed if she is dizzy or weak or cannot stand during a contraction.

There will be times in labor when you will have to insist on your wife's doing things when she strongly disagrees with you. Staying in bed may be one of the first. As labor progresses, her udgment may well become clouded. You, on the other hand, are able to see things from a less subjective perspective. For while you are helping her with labor, she is going through it. You will need to be firm, but not bossy. More than anything she needs your support. But you need cool logic, and you must precisely execute what you have learned.

As labor coach in the labor room, you will continue the record keeping job that you began at home. You will also be making strenuous efforts to keep your wife comfortable by helping her change position, by wiping her face with a cool face cloth, by keeping her lips moist, by massaging her back or legs. You will need to be especially alert for signs of tension. As time goes on, your wife will have to work harder to concentrate. Not only will the contractions become stronger, but her energy will be lessening.

You will have the important job of combining the conditioning you have practiced at home with kind words in between contractions about what a good job she is doing. This is the time when your practice will show results. You will have only to say "Relax" or to touch a tense part and your wife will respond. She will be working hard, but so will you.

Mood changes

As labor progresses, you will find that your wife's mood will change. She will become all business. Chit-chat between contractions will disappear. In fact, talking may well irritate her. You would do well to remain alert for this. It is a sign that your wife is becoming tired. You can help immensely by keeping quiet and going about your job of coach using tactile cues for relaxing.

When your wife *is* irritable, try not to take it personally. She still loves you and knows you are a great help. She also knows that she would be lost without your presence. She knows this only too well if you have been asked to step out for whatever reason and she has had a contraction. Nevertheless, the effort of coping with labor is so great that her resources are shrinking. And verbal abuse is a form of tension release. Usually, the last kind of irritable behavior rears its ugly head about the time of transition.

You would do well to get a progress report from the doctor if you possibly can. It is truly amazing the renewed energy that appears in a woman near exhaustion when she learns how close she is to her goal—the birth of the baby.

Keeping staff informed

As labor coach, you have a responsibility to keep everyone informed. Your wife, your doctor, and the hospital staff will rely on you for any information you can supply. You are an important member of the obstetrical team. And as with any team it works best through mutual cooperation. Communication is the key to effective team cooperation. After all, everyone is basically interested in the well-being of your wife and baby.

What needs to be communicated is that you have a job to do that does not interfere with the jobs of any of the other members of this team. Your image should be projected as one of competent control of the situation with respect for the other team members and their functions. This means that you and your wife must demonstrate by your actions that you are working together effectively.

Vocabulary of labor

You must also know the vocabulary of the labor and delivery room so you can understand when the other team members give you a progress report. For example, if you ask a doctor who examines your wife, "How is she doing?" he will most likely answer "Fine" and let it go at that. If however you say, "How many centimeters is she dilated?" before he has a chance to think about it, he will automatically answer, "About three centimeters." When he does think about it, he will realize that you are a man who talks his language. You may get even more information than you request.

Communicating with the hospital nursing staff is equally important. Remember, these are people in a helping profession. With you in the room doing the things they usually do to make women in labor comfortable, many labor room nurses feel left out. This means that you have to make extra efforts to be polite and tactful with them. They still have the essential function of monitoring your wife and baby. They will be coming into the room at regular intervals to take your wife's blood pressure and listen to the baby's heartbeat.

This is a time for you to show that you are not trying to be Mr. Top Banana. Offer whatever information you have and ask how your wife and baby are doing. If the nurse comes in during a contraction, do not tell her dogmatically that she has to wait. Of course, as labor coach it is your job to run interference. But you can get her to wait by distracting her, by explaining what your wife is doing. In other words, be diplomatic. You may want her help. It will be a lot easier to get if she thinks you are a nice, cooperative husband rather than a bossy so-and-so who is keeping her from getting her work done.

HELPING WITH TECHNIQUES

Of all the things you have to do as labor coach, helping your wife with the techniques is the most vital. Without them she would be lost to the forces of labor. In fact, for one reason or another, most women do lose one or more contractions during the process of labor. This is not a shortcoming on their part, nor does it mean that they have not practiced enough. Being distracted or being examined may be enough for your wife to miss the beginning of a contraction. If the contraction gets away from her, it is very difficult, almost impossible, to catch up to it. It only has to happen once or twice for her to realize how well PPM works to control her perception of pain. She will then be even more determined to concentrate.

In early labor, your job is pretty easy. You time contractions and check for relaxation. You encourage your wife to put off using any breathing techniques until she really needs something for control. As long as she can talk or laugh during a contraction, it would be premature to begin any special breathing.

Slow ryhthmic breathing

When your wife does feel the need for control, she should begin slow rhythmic chest breathing. She can do this in any position. You can help her by being sure she is relaxed and actually breathing slowly. Remember, slow rhythmic chest breathing is supposed to be a relaxed extension of normal breathing, taking place in the chest instead of using the abdominal muscles. Following the breathing basics—focus eyes, think "chest," relax all muscles not being used—and making an effort to concentrate are usually enough to give your wife control through this period of her labor. Yet many women do become tense. This is a reaction to wanting labor to be here and over.

Be alert for signs of tension. Use the verbal cues you practiced together. It will be especially helpful to you as her coach to get her into the habit of responding to your cues as early as possible in labor. In this way, when she really needs your help under the stress of real labor you will have established the response.

Many intelligent people fall into the trap of seeing the whole labor process and psychoprophylaxis as another intellectual exercise to be added to their repertoire. You must make every effort to avoid this pitfall. Labor is real. It will be happening to your wife. The only way the two of you can control the situation is by the automatic responses you develop in practice and can execute with precision, as a team in labor.

Adding effleurage

As the contractions increase in intensity, your wife will want more tools for control. When slow rhythmic chest breathing is no longer enough by itself, it is time to add the effleurage. This will give her another activity to be coordinated with the breathing she is doing in response to the sensations she perceives. Many women find this combination effective enough to carry them through most of labor.

As labor coach, it is your duty to observe your wife's reactions. Compare her relaxation during contractions with the practice sessions you worked at together at home. You will be watching for the little signs—tense fingers, knitted eyebrows, stiffly held head. When you do see a sign of tension, take action. No speeches. Gently touch or stroke the tense area. Say softly but firmly: "Relax."

Working together

Remember you are working together. Your wife needs to know that you will take care of those things that she misses. But she also needs to know that you know she is doing many things well.

If you think she is having some difficulty, say so. And say it right after the contraction. You might say: "That seemed like a hard contraction. How are you doing?" If she thinks she is doing well, great. Let her continue as she is doing. If she also thought it was a hard one or that she did not have good control, see if you both think the next one is as hard. After the next one, if needed, you can suggest adding another tool or switching to a more complex breathing technique.

Whatever you decide, the important thing is that you have let your wife know in the most tangible way that you are in there pulling with her. You are telling her, in effect, that you know how hard she is working and that you are trying to make it as smooth as possible for her. Always approach a subject with her in a positive way. Look for the things you can compliment first before you make any suggestions or criticisms.

Above all, never under any circumstances let yourself get frustrated and say something you will regret like: "You are doing everything wrong." She is not, of course, doing everything wrong. In all probability she is doing most things right. What has happened is that you think it should be different, more like the teacher demonstrated in class or more like you practiced at home. But this is labor. And that statement can shatter your wife's confidence. Any coach who would say that is more concerned with his own importance as a coach than he is with his wife's welfare.

The labor coach is present to provide advice, suggestions, and support. He is supposed to use his objectivity, coupled with his personal involvement and knowledge of PPM to provide an atmosphere in which the laboring woman, his wife, can take an active part in the dignified, reasonably comfortable progress of her labor. You can best fulfill your duties as a coach by helping your wife to cope with each contraction as it occurs.

The beauty of using PPM is the flexibility of the method in actual practice. Your training and practice is exact. You learned to an automatic level the complex patterns of behavior that are the tools your wife can use. When they are put into use in labor, it is with the pragmatic understanding of using whatever works best. Many women find that slow rhythmic chest breathing with effleurage can keep them in control throughout most of labor. Other women switch to shallow breathing midway. Still others use both and choose to return to slow chest breathing later in labor.

There are no hard and fast rules about what must be used at any one point in labor nor in what sequence the techniques must be employed. The good labor coach is the one who can make suggestions concerning techniques based on his observations of how effective the tool being used at the moment is in providing the woman with 1) adequate cerebral stimulation, 2) adequate control of the situation, and 3) adequate opportunity to relax during contractions to prevent fatigue.

Counting off contractions

As the contractions themselves last longer, in addition to your observations, you should be counting off the contractions in ten to fifteen second intervals. This will help your wife by making the duration seem shorter as you call it off in segments.

Continue to remind your wife to empty her bladder. She will probably not think of it herself. Offer her the bedpan between contractions. If you have an aversion to handling the bedpan, offer it to your wife and then seek the nurse and tell her your wife needs assistance to come off.

At this time your wife will definitely not be allowed to eat or to drink large amounts of fluid. She will probably feel dry in the mouth. Most doctors will permit ice chips, if available. Certainly frequent mouth rinses would help even if only with plain water. If she does not find the flavor unpleasant, the sugar in the lollipops may also be helpful at this time.

As the work of coping with each contraction requires increasing amounts of concentration, your wife will want to use the time in between contractions to rest. She may even sleep. However, if labor has been unusually long or if your wife had little rest before it began, the doctor may want to give her an analgesic to help her relax. Do not be alarmed; he is not trying to "knock her out." Many obstetricians who regularly practice PPM find that a small dose of analgesic given judiciously can enhance the woman's efforts and extend her ability to withstand the desire to give up.

This is a time when your presence as a coach is particularly needed. The effect of the analgesic that is desired is to assist your wife to relax totally between contractions without interfering with the progress of labor. This means that while she will be awake during contractions, she may be somewhat dopey when labor begins. You can help by being alert for the beginning of each contraction. Place your hand lightly on the top of her abdomen. When you feel it begin to tighten, you say, "Contraction begins." You take a deep breath with her and if necessary breathe with her during the contraction. This will help her to stay on top of the contractions instead of letting them get ahead of her.

THE PERIOD OF TRANSITION

The most difficult part of labor is the shortest. Transition is the period when the cervix is not completely dilated but the baby's head is far enough down into the birth canal to create the pressure that gives your wife the urge to push. During transition, you can expect your wife to be nauseated and if she has anything in her stomach, she will vomit. She may experience chills and/or have cold extremities. And she probably will have uncontrollable trembling, especially of the large muscles in her legs. It is a time when it will be difficult for her to communicate and almost impossible to relax. This is where you come in.

After a contraction where you recognize any or many of these symptoms, tell your wife that you think it is transition and that you are going to get a doctor to examine her. He will do an internal examination and confirm or deny your interpretation.

Be sure you wait until after the contraction is over. This is the time your wife will especially need your assistance during each contraction. Because it is difficult for her to concentrate, she will need you to remind her to relax. The contractions themselves are so erratic, it will take every ounce of her energy just to stay on top. Be positive. Tell her how close she is. Point out that you know how hard it is for her to cope but that she has done so well for so long and labor is almost over.

When the doctor examines your wife, he will be determining how far dilated her cervix is. If he finds that the cervix is eight to nine centimeters, he will tell her not to push. You can be a big help. Stay beside your wife constantly. The contractions will be long—from sixty to ninety seconds—with more than one peak and with strong, intermittant urges to push. She will barely have time to recover in between as the interval may be as little as thirty seconds from the end of one until the beginning of the next. To help her to relax, encourage her to do slow rhythmic chest breathing in between contractions. Breathe with her during contractions if necessary to help her start on top and stay there.

Counteracting urge of push

Be alert for any signs that she is feeling the urge to push. This might be a sudden overall tensing of her body, or a grunting noise, or a cessation of the breathing techniques to verbalize. As soon as you see this say: "Blow . . . blow . . . blow . . . blow . . . ." She will blow in short hard bursts until the urge passes. Much of pushing is an involuntary muscular reaction to the internal pressures which nobody can really control. The purpose of this breathing sequence is to eliminate the additional pressure created by the voluntary effort.

Do not relax during a contraction. The urge to push may reappear at any time during the contraction. The unpredictability of it makes these contractions hard to control. Have your wife keep up the pant-blow rhythm interrupting it with consecutive blowing for the urge until the contraction subsides. When your wife takes her deep breath at the end of the contraction, encourage her to continue doing slow rhythmic chest breathing. This will be accompanied by her concentration on relaxing. It will be an automatic adjunct to her breathing by this time in labor. Slow rhythmic chest breathing also forces her to assume a more normal breathing pattern.

Your wife will probably be very negative and discouraged

during this phase of labor. Try to bolster her spirits. Keep reminding her that she will be able to push soon and then the baby will be here. One ingenious husband brought along a baby outfit and whipped it out at the moment his wife was ready to give up. She rallied with remarkable vigor.

PERMISSION TO PUSH

The doctor will be nearby and he will reexamine your wife to determine her progress. As soon as he feels the cervix is fully dilated, he will grant her permission to push. Two things will happen. First, your wife will experience a tremendous sense of relief at being allowed to push. The act of pushing is a positive action she can take; completely the opposite of the holding back during transition. And second, the quality of the contractions will change. They will revert to the much less trying pattern of building to a peak, maintaining it, and declining. This is the pattern that your wife controlled so well in active labor.

Your role in the labor room when your wife has been given permission to push is definite. You are to be sure that the bed is lowered and that your wife is resting on two pillows—one under her shoulders and the other the long way under her head and extending down her back.

As the contraction begins, you are to call out the mechanics and signals for pushing: "Breathe in . . . breathe out . . . breathe in . . . breathe out . . . breathe in . . . hold it. Round shoulders . . . elbows out . . . relax perineum . . . push. Keep it up . . . keep it up . . . keep it up."

If you are to be supporting your wife's legs, you should be standing beside her at about knee level so that when she raises her legs, you can support one on your shoulder and the other with your arm. She should renew her breath without releasing the muscles engaged in pushing at about ten to fifteen seconds. If she looks red in the face, you might encourage her by saying:

"Let it out . . . don't stop pushing . . . take another breath. Push . . . push . . . keep it up. That's good."

In between contractions you will find that your wife is a changed woman. She is exhilarated and full of questions. There is again a rest interval of from two to five minutes between contractions. You will both be feeling the excitement of almost being there. If you can, encourage your wife to breathe deeply and slowly in between contractions and to relax.

Patch of head

Most doctors will have women delivering first babies push in the labor room until a patch of the baby's head about the size of a quarter can be seen during the contraction at the vaginal opening. Since you will be in a position to see it first, tell your wife. You will see the opening widen and a patch of dark wetness push forward. Do not worry. You will not be delivering your own baby. It will slip back as soon as she stops pushing. But do share it with her. She is working at the most exhausting physical exertion she will ever do. Reward her at every opportunity with news of the progress which she is making.

At this point, the doctor will make plans to move your wife to the delivery room. In most hospitals this means that she will be assisted to a stretcher that is the same height as the bed. She will be wheeled down the hall to the delivery room. And, in the delivery room, she will be assisted over to the delivery table. All of this will hopefully be accomplished in between contractions. However, if a contraction occurs, your wife should be prepared to blow as she did during transition as she cannot push effectively while in transit and it is better to allow just the natural body forces to work until she can get into proper position. It will probably be for only one, or possibly two, contractions.

It is quite likely that you will miss this maneuver. Many doctors who are accustomed to working with prepared couples will take the father along to scrub and have his gown changed for the delivery room. This gives the doctor the opportunity for any last minute instructions and the father the opportunity for any last minute questions. If your doctor does not feel that this is necessary and leaves you with your wife, coach her just as you did in transition.

Do not interfere with the transferring of your wife to or from the stretcher. The nurses are trained in proper body mechanics. If you attempt to push or pull leaning over a bed or stretcher you have a pretty good chance of spasming muscles along your back giving yourself a terrible backache from the strain. Besides, your wife is perfectly capable of sliding over from one surface to another. Your job is to remind her to blow when she feels the urge to push.

VARIATIONS IN NORMAL LABOR

At this point you have for all intents reached the end of labor and begun delivery. The cervix is completely dilated, virtually disappeared, and your baby is on the verge of being born.

The discussion thus far has dealt with the anticipated progress of normal labor. There are a number of variations, still within the range of *normal* labor, of which you should be aware so that you can help your wife cope with any one should it occur.

Hyperventilation

The simplest variation is rather a superficial one and can be corrected easily by your efforts as labor coach. It is called hyperventilation. That long word describes a state of imbalance caused by improper breathing. When the exhalation or out-breath is longer than the inhalation, or in-breath, the body loses carbon dioxide at a rate that is too fast. The result is that your wife will report that she feels dizzy or has tingling sensations in her hands or feet or around her mouth.

These unpleasant sensations can be relieved by rebreathing

exhaled air. This is the reason you brought the small paper bag. If you cannot locate the bag at the appropriate moment, simply have your wife cup both hands so that the pinkies lie side by side and place both hands over her nose and mouth and breathe into them. This will accomplish the same thing.

Hyperventilation has often been pointed to by critics of prepared childbirth. They claim that hyperventilation causes changes in the mother's blood gases which interfere with the baby's oxygen supply. Prolonged hyperventilation may do exactly that. But in the properly prepared woman, the symptoms are recognized early and corrected.

It is in the unprepared woman where the real danger lies. She hyperventilates in fear, the resulting sensations create more fear because she cannot understand what is happening. Her response is to become more agitated which in turn causes her to breathe even more erratically. In the extreme, hyperventilation can cause such severe chemical imbalance that it results in spasming of muscles including the uterus. This can be a real danger to the baby.

Each contraction during labor temporarily reduces the blood supply to the baby. After all, blood vessels are really only tubes. When the uterus contracts, it squeezes all the tubes that pass through it. These contractions usually last around a minute or less. It is like holding your breath for a minute. But if the uterus contracts and does not relax, the oxygen supply to the baby is cut off. This is a tragic situation which may require emergency measures. Luckily it is a rare occurrence. And the prepared couple are in the best position to prevent it by reestablishing proper breathing.

Hyperventilation should not occur at all in the prepared woman if she is doing the breathing techniques properly. It does occur if deep breathing is done too rapidly or if shallow breathing is not shallow enough. These are the two main things you should look for in actual labor. The tendency is to speed up all breathing because labor is a tension-making situation. Your job is to minimize the tension by providing calm, reassuring instructions.

Time your wife's breathing, as well as the contractions. If she is breathing too fast, she is tense. Slow her down. Talk about it between contractions. If need be, breathe with her for the rest of the contraction. Be especially alert for the proper technique when the changeover is made from slow rhythmic breathing to shallow breathing.

Shallow means very high in the chest. It is easy to get sloppy and think that the breathing is high when really it has moved only midway up in the chest. What happens then is that the rate is much too fast for the depth, and this is a time hyperventilation can easily occur. Watch for signs that shallow breathing is really high.

If you see your wife's bosom moving up and down with each breath, she is not breathing high enough. Get in the habit during practice sessions of checking to see where your wife is breathing. Periodically check rate during practice periods. Remember, it is natural to speed up in labor.

It is best to prevent hyperventilation. This requires teamwork both before and during labor. And it also requires the constant attention of the labor coach and his precision in maintaining the proper breathing patterns.

Induction

Another normal variation in labor occurs with assistance from the outside. For some women, labor does not progress smoothly. It may continue for many hours making slow progress, or it may move in unpredictable patterns of fast progress and then no progress for long periods.

Your obstetrician will be monitoring the progress of labor. It is unreasonable to expect him to sit and hold your wife's hand throughout labor. But he will be in constant communication with the hospital staff once she has been admitted. If for any reason he feels that labor is not moving along as it should, and this is a decision he makes based on medical knowledge and his experience, he will prescribe a drug which will implement the labor.

This drug is much like the chemical called oxytocin which is secreted by your wife's pituitary gland. Oxytocin controls labor. Some women do not secrete sufficient amounts of this chemical to keep labor moving. By administering this chemical, the doctor is providing artificial stimulation to bring about regular uterine contractions that will make labor more effective.

This is in no way a reflection on the woman. She would be able to deliver the baby on her own eventually. But by engaging the services of a competent and sympathetic obstetrician, you have provided your wife with the opportunity to have this baby with the maximum amount of comfort and, in this case, in a much shorter time.

Your job as labor coach will be an especially trying one once induction (another way of saying implementation) is begun. Oxytocin may be given in a number of ways. It may be administered by an injection, a suppository, or a lozenge that is melted in the mouth. It depends much on what is available in your hospital and the route your doctor prefers. The above information is given only so that you will be aware of the possibilities. It is not given for you to make a choice. That is your physician's decision.

Once oxytocin is given, you must be on your toes. Within a few minutes, your wife's labor will intensify dramatically. You need to be at her side and prepared to get right into a more complex technique than she has been using. The first changed contraction will undoubtedly catch her by surprise. Even if she knows that labor is going to accelerate with induction, that first contraction thereafter will seem so much stronger than previous ones that she may even lose it before she can get on top. Your job is to get her back on the path. Labor will probably progress rapidly. What might have taken several hours may happen in only two. Be alert for signs of transition as labor progresses. Because labor moves so much more quickly, it can be exhausting and overwhelming for your wife. Be sure to stay nearby. Offer to rub her back.

If oxytocin has been given by intravenous infusion, your wife may be reluctant to use her arm. This is a normal fear even though most intravenous sites are now chosen to allow for complete mobility. Offer to do her effleurage. Your presence will be extremely important to her ability to cope. As with unassisted labor, your wife will need permission to push and will probably push in the labor room first.

Induction has received a great deal of publicity as a way of having a baby by appointment. It should be mentioned here that while this does sound convenient, it does not always work. Many women go into labor on their own before their appointment. Some women are not ready for labor even by the appointment date. It is useless to try induction unless the woman's cervix is ready to make the changes that occur in labor. All that will happen then is a flurry of hard contractions that force the baby's head against a closed cervix. It would be much wiser to wait for labor to begin naturally.

Posterior presentation

Another variation in labor, caused by the position that the baby can take, is called a posterior presentation. This means that the baby's head is down but instead of the top of his head pointing forward, the baby is lying so that the top or hardest part of his head is pointed backwards. As a result of this backward pressure, the labor is experienced in the lower back or lumbosacral region, rather than primarily in the lower abdomen. This is called back labor.

Because the contractions are felt in the back, relief from them needs to be directed toward that area. Your wife will have to consciously work at relaxing the area. She should deliberately think of each component over and over: Relax back, buttocks, thighs. She should continue using the breathing techniques to provide her mind with a complex pattern to execute.

You can provide counterpressure. You can do this by balling your fists and pushing them into your wife's lower back on either side of her spine. When your arms get tired, you can kneel one knee on the edge of the bed and have her lie with her lower back hard against it.

Some women find sitting tailor fashion most comfortable. It puts the weight of the baby forward and on the bed, and does relieve the pressure. Sitting can be combined with counterpressure. This is where your tennis balls come into play. Roll the bed as far upright as it will go. Place each tennis ball where you would place your fists if she were side-lying—that is, at the lower back on each side of the spine. This combination is quite effective as it provides the maximum relief with the minimum effort. The upright bed provides a backrest and support for your wife. Her weight as she leans back will provide the counterpressure of the tennis balls.

Back labor is the most exhausting of all labor variations. The reason for this is that the other forms of labor remain intermittent requiring intense concentration for short periods of time. Back labor is only partially intermittent. While back pressure crescendos with each contraction, it does not completely subside in between. The residual backache becomes a chronic irritant to the woman. She must work throughout each contraction and possibly between to relax the lower back and thighs, as well as trying to maintain overall relaxation of her other muscle groups. For this reason, you must make special attempts to think of every trick you can to help your wife conserve energy.

Use the bed and pillows to support her limbs and head in any position she finds comfortable. Avoid taxing her by unnecessary conversation, although it will help her immensely if you talk to her throughout each contraction. She may find it comforting to have you stroke her thighs and legs between contractions. Your role is extremely important with back labor. Your presence and support can make it possible for your wife to cope with what is essentially a normal labor.

Posterior presentation is normal. The baby can and should be born vaginally. But back labor is uncomfortable and exhausting. In this instance the presence of a prepared father can make or break the experience for his wife. You need to understand that back labor is happening and then use your head. Your goals are to make your wife as comfortable as possible and to conserve her energy.

Back labor is a variation of normal labor. It should not be confused with back pressure that most women feel in the beginning of labor. Back pressure, often described as backache, will change as labor progresses. It will become a starting point for the early contractions that begin in the lower back and then radiate forward. As the intensity of the contractions grows, the importance of back pressure diminishes. In true back labor, this does not happen. Contractions begin and end in the lower back. You might look for this differentiation in your wife's early labor. If you suspect she is having back labor, consult your obstetrician. He can verify the baby's presentation—a subject that your wife may not have discussed with him.

DELIVERY VARIATIONS

In addition to the variations of labor, there are two variations of delivery that the prepared parents should know about. The first variation is the result of normal differences that occur within women. It is called breech delivery. All that this means is that instead of the baby's head being born first, his bottom will precede him. There is no danger to the baby since he does not breathe until all of him is born. Many parents fear the baby will drown if his head is not born first. This just is not true!

The obstetrician can usually tell when he does his internal examination which end of the baby is down. It is possible that a baby who is in the breech position at the beginning of labor will rotate during labor, but this is not too likely. However, there is no reason in the world why the position of the baby should interfere with your working together in labor and delivery.

The only thing to remember is that labor will probably be somewhat longer. This is quite logical if you realize that the baby is making a path for himself by moving soft tissue out of his way. If he is pushing his hard head through soft tissue, it is apt to move and stretch quite easily. However, if he is pressing onward with his soft baby bottom, the going will be a little slower. So, your job as labor coach will be primarily to make every effort to conserve your wife's energy.

Caesarian section

The other variation is surgical. Many women are faced with the necessity of having their babies by Caesarian section (C/S). Historically named for Julius Caesar, who was born by a primitive version of this surgical procedure, Caesarian sectioning is major abdominal surgery. It is usually performed for one of two reasons. Either the baby is too large to fit through its mother's bony pelvis or the baby during the process of labor is in distress and must be born immediately or die. In each case, there is no choice. The risk of major surgery is outweighed by the danger to the mother and baby if it is not done.

Most women who are told that they have a small pelvis and may have to have a C/S are also told that because surgery is always a risk, they will be given an opportunity for trial labor. That is, they will be given the chance of trying to deliver the baby vaginally. This means that they will be going into labor. It means that if the baby is just small enough to slip through, surgery will not be necessary.

No promises are made. It is understood that it is nobody's fault if labor proves that the baby is just too big to fit. But what it does mean is that this woman is going to go into labor and needs to be just as well prepared as the woman who expects to deliver vaginally all along. She will have to cope with contractions, and she will need just as much encouragement and support. Perhaps she needs a little more. Because even though nobody says it out loud there is a threat over her head: if this does not work, you are going to have an operation. That in itself is pretty scary.

Your job as labor coach is to act as though you believe that the two of you are going all the way together. Your wife needs your strength. The things you need to do are the same as if you were expecting a vaginal delivery—keep a record of labor, make your wife comfortable, and help her with the controlled relaxation and breathing techniques. You may be called on to do more to keep her spirits up. Even if the doctor does decide that the baby must be delivered by C/S, you will find that both of you feel that you worked together and gave it your best efforts. It is this positive feeling that pervades the prepared experience and underlines how important a couple really are to each other.

There is often little or no warning for the woman who must be delivered by C/S. Once in the hospital, both mother and baby are monitored frequently. The nurse will take your wife's blood pressure and listen to the baby's heartbeat. This is really the only indicator from the outside that all is going well with the baby. However, should there be any problem with the baby's heartbeat—either too fast or too slow—the doctor will be called in to check. He will look for other signs that the baby is in distress. If he feels that this is the situation, it immediately becomes an emergency.

The physician will discuss the situation with you. If he feels that the baby is in grave danger, your wife will be anesthetized and the baby delivered by C/S. There are any number of reasons why this can occur. Some have to do with internal environment. Others have to do with the labor itself. Fortunately, emergency Caesarian-sections are rare, but thank goodness for their availability when needed.

Since the mother who has an emergency C/S is not forewarned that this will happen, she can use all the tools of prepared childbirth up until the time that she is informed that surgery is required. There is no change in the role of the labor coach either. The operation is unforeseen. You need only know that it is there to save the lives of your wife and baby if needed. It is one of the real reasons for using the services of a competent obstetrician in a hospital setting. Despite all the drawbacks of today's hospitals, financial and emotional, there is a singular advantage of having all the equipment and personnel on standby just in case *your* wife or *your* baby needs them.

4

In the Delivery Room

The presence of fathers in the delivery room has caused a controversy that has received much publicity. The cause of the notoriety is blurred because it cannot be traced to any one single factor. Professionals as a group tend to be conservative. Interested in the welfare of the mother and the baby, they are often not informed about the role of the PPM-trained husband and the importance of his being present. They have, in fact, been taking care of mothers and babies very well for many years and need to be persuaded that the presence of the father will not increase their responsibilities and work.

Fathers, in the past, have done their part in keeping the gulf between themselves and the professionals wide. By being demanding or by belligerently disregarding the instructions of professionals, fathers themselves have helped to foster an unfavorable image among the staffs of hospital obstetrical units.

Another gray area that may influence the acceptance of the husband as a member of the obstetrical team lies in the realm of physician-patient relationship. Obstetricians are often the recipients of a kind of transference. That is, many women "fall in love" with their obstetricians and endow them with an aura of greatness for a period after confinement. With couples who have worked together to deliver this child of theirs, this transference still takes place, but the recipient is the husband. It requires a mature individual to be able to relinquish the personal satisfaction that comes from being so highly regarded in order to provide his patient with the most meaningful support he can — her husband.

This is another reason you are urged to interview physicians and choose one carefully. If the doctor is unsure of what the father's role is supposed to be, he may see the father's presence as an implied criticism of his own ability to perform, or he may feel that his professional judgment is being called into question. As this is not your intention, you must communicate with the doctor from the earliest time possible during the prenatal period.

It is not wise to accept a physician on a personal recommendation if he does not endorse the kind of labor and delivery experience you and your wife are seeking. Many couples do, with the intention of trying to convince him, only to find themselves sadly disappointed at the crucial time of delivery. It is unrealistic to expect to argue rationally with a physician who has revealed that he has high emotional stakes in the controversy.

This is not an indictment of the medical and paramedical professionals. It is meant to reveal one fact that is often overlooked by the general public. Doctors and nurses are people first. They are just as subject to their own prejudices as are other people. They choose to work in situations which are comfortable for them. If you as a father make their situation uncomfortable, they will oppose you. Therefore, for your own well-being try to choose a situation which is compatible with your goals.

Many of the hospitals which allow husbands in the delivery room have come to this liberal point of view because of public pressure. This being a free enterprise society, financial support or withdrawal is the strongest weapon the public can wield.

People seek out medical care that is in keeping with their needs and desires. If a doctor or hospital does not provide the style of care they are seeking, they look elsewhere. In this way, the public wishes are made known.

It does not take a hospital board of businessmen long to realize that their policy regarding husbands in the delivery room is a pivotal issue when prospective parents register their positions and withdraw their support if the delivery room is closed to the husband. This is the kind of pressure that will eventually change hospital policies. Your opposition will weigh in favor of change but probably not in time for you to take advantage of it.

There are a number of standard arguments against the presence of husbands in the delivery room. It may be of some help to you to know what they are and why they are not valid when applied to the prepared father.

1) Husbands will faint in the delivery room.

This argument has great legal implications and weighs heavily with the hospital review board. Many argue that the sight of the delivery will frighten the father who does not have medical education. He will become faint, fall, and injure himself in the delivery room. This may be the case with the unprepared father, but is highly unlikely with the father who has attended classes.

The prepared father knows essentially what to expect. He has seen slides of an actual delivery and, possibly, a motion picture. In addition, the prepared father has specific tasks to do. He is there to help his wife. He should be sitting on a stool directly behind her head or immediately to one side or the other. He is *not* there as an idle sightseer. He is a part of the procedure.

Obstetricians who are familiar with prepared couples know how to use the husband to relay messages. This father is so involved in what is happening that it is less likely that he will faint than it is that a nursing or medical student merely observing will faint. In fact, there has been more documentation to substantiate the latter than there has been to prove that fainting fathers are a reality.

2) Fathers in the delivery room will increase infection.

This is a fear of pediatricians who are responsible for the welfare of the babies in the nursery. However, it is based on conjecture. It would seem that professionals expect fathers to be so stupid that they cannot follow simple instructions.

The prepared father is gowned and masked. He has been told not to touch any of the equipment or sterile drapes covering his wife. With these admonitions, he is ready to assume his position beside his wife and offer her his support. Those hospitals which regularly permit fathers in the delivery room may also expect him to scrub his hands before he puts on a fresh gown and mask for the delivery. Therefore, if there is any increase in the incidence of infection, it is unlikely to be caused by the presence of a prepared father in the delivery room.

3) The delivery room is hectic. We do not have personnel to supervise husbands.

The delivery room personnel, particularly the nurses, are extremely busy with the many technical tasks surrounding the delivery of the baby. Because they may not understand the place or the function of the prepared father in the delivery room, they incorrectly assume his activity will require their attention.

The prepared father is not just another person in the delivery room. Most professionals are accustomed to having extra people —medical or nursing students—present in the delivery room for the purpose of seeing a baby being born. Although viewing childbirth may be an exciting side attraction, this is not the purpose of the prepared father's being present. He is there to help his wife participate in the birth of their baby. He has a position at her head. He has tasks to assist her with the explusive effort. He is not standing over the obstetrician's shoulder as the usual observers are. He is not wandering around the delivery room for a better point of view.

There is no need for additional personnel to supervise prepared fathers. They learn their role from their instructor and in most cases carry it out with precision.

4) Husbands will not understand what the obstetrician is doing and will physically assault the doctor.

Both during and after delivery, good obstetrical practice dictates that the physician handle and examine the woman's genitalia and internal organs. For some reason, in some quarters, it is expected that husbands who are present will consider it improper and attack the physician. This claim can only be interpreted as an emotional shortcoming on the part of the person who would make such a statement. That person must consider the procedure improper or he would not expect the attack.

The prepared father is informed about delivery. There is no reason to suppose that he would object to any one part of the medical care. There is even less reason to anticipate the husband's attacking a professional who is offering care to his wife.

What has happened is that professionals have extended the notion of privacy beyond reasonable limits. While they consider it perfectly normal for a couple to copulate to create a baby, they see it as perverse if the husband is present during delivery or even during a medical examination. This kind of reasoning can work a great deprivation on the woman who wants and needs her husband's support, as well as on the husband who needs to know that basically, even if uncomfortable, his wife is all right. The resources of the prepared couple should never be underestimated or undermined.

5) What if something goes wrong?

There is always the possibility during any delivery that something can happen which will require obstetrical intervention. Prepared husbands are aware of this, and as part of their preparation they are trained to follow the directions of their obstetrician. If the physician feels that the husband can no longer be of assistance to his wife, the husband will be asked to leave.

In class, it has been emphasized that there are situations, though rare, which can arise which will require the particular skills of the obstetrician. If the father is asked to leave, he is expected to do so immediately and without an argument. Usually, the doctor will ask the father to leave if it is necessary to anesthetize his wife.

Some doctors permit the husband to stay until his wife is under the anesthesia, so that she can benefit from his presence as long as possible. But once she is anesthetized, there is no job for the husband, no reason for him to be there except as a sightseer. This is the time he can have physical problems. It is therefore best if he does leave the delivery room.

If, however, the baby has a birth defect and all else seems normal, most physicians who practice PPM agree that it is most helpful to the couple if they remain together. Husband and wife can support each other. They both know exactly what is happening. Each knows that the other knows what the situation is and that he does not have to face telling the other at a later time. This can be of immeasurable value. Husband and wife can then jointly focus their attention on the welfare of their baby.

"What if . . ." is perhaps the biggest reason given for barring husbands from the delivery room. It is truly unfortunate because the woman needs the comfort and support of her husband in an emergency even more than during normal labor and delivery. Yet, because many professionals feel personally responsible for any problem no matter how naturally it occurs, they expect recriminations from parents who are aware of the emergency. This is far from the truth. Parents allowed to be together to comfort each other and to watch the care being offered to their child are grateful and supportive of the professionals no matter what the outcome. It is usually the parents who do not know what has happened who have doubts. So, the "what if . . ." arguments are also invalid for keeping fathers from the delivery room.

Information: your best armament

The best armament you as a prospective father can have for your experience in the delivery room is adequate information. You need to know exactly what to expect. You need to know what is happening to your wife, what you are to be doing, and where you are to be doing it.

Once your wife has been moved into the delivery room, you will be surprised how different things will seem to you. Instead of the feeling of distant anticipation that has been with you for most of labor, you will feel the excitement of knowing that the baby is practically here.

This sensation will be emphasized by the electric atmosphere of the delivery room. The nurses will be bustling around placing equipment within the doctor's reach. They will be making sure that your wife is in a good position on the delivery table and properly draped with sterile covers.

EQUIPMENT IN DELIVERY ROOM

When you took your tour of the hospital and saw the delivery room, you probably never envisioned it as it appears when you actually arrive there for business. The equipment may seem bewildering or even frightening.

There will be, of course, the delivery table on which your wife will be lying. When you see it on the tour, it may look like a big metal table with thin cushions on top and several levers on each side. While it was flat when your wife slid onto it, the table does not stay that way. Stirrups, which are leg rests that support your wife's lower legs and knees, are added to each side at about the height of your wife's hips. Your wife is assisted into the stirrups so that she is lying flat to her hips and then her legs are raised and supported. The part of the table that was under her legs when she was lying completely flat, folds down so that the doctor can actually stand right at the scene of the action. Once in the proper position on the delivery table, your wife is then covered from the waist down with sterile sheets, leaving exposed only the actual birth area.

It will be helpful to your wife if her wrists are free so that she can grasp the handgrip or stirrup support when she is pushing. It is customary in most hospitals to restrain a woman's hands with leather cuffs attached to the sides of the delivery table. It is not painful, and it serves to keep her from reaching into the delivery area and inadvertantly contaminating the procedure or interfering with the doctor. This is really only a problem when a woman is under the influence of heavy sedation and cannot control the involuntary urge to touch the stretching vaginal tissue.

The prepared woman expects these sensations and knows that she is not to touch the sterile drapes or reach for the baby. Therefore, check to see that your wife's hands are free. If they are not, ask the doctor if they may be as it will help her with pushing. If they are already free, remind her to keep them loosely on the handgrip or stirrup support which will be within easy reach when she is in the relaxed position. In this way, she will not have to begin searching for a handhold when the next contraction begins, and there will be no danger of her accidentally contaminating the sterile field.

Also in the delivery room is a piece of equipment which for some reason is disturbing for many people. This is the overhead light. A huge, oversized relative of the dentist's round light, the one in the delivery room hangs from the ceiling and looks like something from the future. It really is an effective way of getting maximum light on a particular area, but it surely is a scary thing for people who are not used to it.

In addition to the equipment for the actual delivery, there is usually equipment ready to receive the baby. A crib is waiting. A delivery room crib is usually a small metal box, covered with a thin mattress ready to receive the baby for a short period immediately after birth. A source of oxygen is nearby so a small mask can be laid near the baby to provide an oxygen enriched environment right after birth. There may be an incubator waiting, too. Do not be alarmed if you see this. It does not mean that there is anything wrong with the baby.

An incubator is only a fancy enclosed crib in which the temperature can be controlled. Many babies at birth have difficulty stabilizing their normal body temperature. After all, being born is a great shock even if you only consider the temperature change. Think how you would feel if you were thrust from an environment with an average temperature of 98.6°F into an environment with an average temperature of 72°F. That is pretty hairy. It is rather like being pushed into the Atlantic Ocean on the first hot day of the summer before the water has begun to warm for the season. The incubator just gives the baby a chance to catch up with the change.

Many hospitals which frequently admit prepared couples have added a mirror in the delivery room for the couple to be able to see the birth from the doctor's point of view without getting in the way. The mirror may be on a stand or hung from the ceiling. However, many are only slightly larger than rear-view mirrors similar to the ones on automobiles, and most are not at the proper angle for either of you to see.

In a quiet time between contractions, if your wife wants to use the mirror, ask if it can be adjusted. Usually you will be given permission to approach the mirror and angle it so that your wife can see the delivery area in it. You are the logical person since the doctor and nurse will be wearing sterile gloves. Sometimes, however, the doctor himself will use a sterile towel to keep from actually touching the mirror and adjust the angle for you.

It is a good idea to check with your wife to be sure that she wants to use the mirror as some women have an aversion to actually watching the birth.

It is also worth your while to make all other necessary provisions for your wife to see. This means that if she wears glasses, she will want them in the delivery room. You may find that late in labor when she is most comfortable lying on her side, she will take her glasses off. You should take charge of them so that you can produce them readily in the delivery room.

It is also a good idea to get an elastic protector, such as athletes use, to be sure that the glasses do not accidentally fall off during your wife's strenuous efforts to push. An elastic protector can be made easily if you can not locate one to purchase. Measure a piece of waistband elastic the distance from earpiece to earpiece of the glasses across the back of your wife's head. The elastic can then be fastened to the earpieces. This will keep the glasses from slipping off.

NATURE OF CONTRACTIONS

It will help you to know what your wife is experiencing so that you can offer her adequate support.

The contractions during this stage, called delivery or expulsion, are strong and long. But they are intermittent, so that while your wife will be working extremely hard with each contraction to help push the baby out, she will have from two to five minutes between contractions to catch her breath and rest. This is hard to realize until you are actually there. But you will find that the rest periods are a time when people talk—your wife may make a comment, you may want to praise her, the doctor may give a progress report or add a touch of humor if he feels that it will help ease tensions. It is like no other medical scene.

By the time she is pushing in the delivery room, the baby's head is actually in the vagina. The vaginal tissue and perineum, that area between the vagina and rectum, must stretch to permit the baby to enter the world. The tissue is somewhat elastic. Although in our civilized culture, unless a woman has had a career that requires a great deal of squatting, it is not stretchy enough. As a result, the expulsion of the baby requires a strenuous pushing effort on her part to assist the perineal tissue to stretch. It is much like a brand new rubber balloon. A new balloon has the potential for expanding, but until it has been expanded for the first time, it is very resistant. So it is with your wife's perineum. The sensation of stretching can be unpleasant. The vaginal and perineal tissues are being literally pushed to their fullest with each contraction. As a result, your wife may feel as though she were going to "split apart." At the same time the tissues have an intense burning sensation.

If it were not for the knowledge that she can almost see her baby at this point, it would be almost impossible to get any woman to push effectively. In fact, largely because there are so many sensations, both visual and tactile, a fair number of women forget the mechanisms of pushing when they are in the delivery room.

Coaching during contractions

This is a point at which you can be of immeasurable help as her coach. To keep her on the track, you need to remember the verbal cues for pushing, just as you practiced them at home. As a contraction begins you say: "Inhale . . . exhale . . . inhale . . . exhale . . . inhale . . . block. Round shoulders . . . elbows out . . . tighten . . . relax . . . push. Keep it up . . . very good . . . keep it up."

Keep your eye on the clock if you can. The most effective pushing for delivery allows the woman to renew her air about every fifteen seconds during the contraction. As the second approaches, you say quickly and firmly: "Let it out . . . inhale . . . push . . . push . . . keep pushing." If she is doing it correctly, she will allow the air to explode out of her lungs, take a new breath and continue pushing without ever releasing her abdominal muscles.

After each contraction, be sure to give a progress report to your wife. This is the hardest physical work she will ever do in her life. To keep up the effort she will need to know that what she is doing, she is doing right, and that by doing it she is going to have a baby shortly. And, indeed, by pushing effectively, by using her voluntary muscles to enhance the work of the uterus, she can shorten the time of the second stage which lasts only until the baby is born.

If you can, try to get your wife to relax in between contractions. She can do this by taking several deep breaths at the end of the contraction or by using controlled relaxation. Do the best you can. This is an exciting time for many women, and your wife may not be able to relax as well as she did in labor.

THE EPISIOTOMY

This is the critical time when your obstetrician will decide whether or not to perform an episiotomy. An episiotomy is a surgical incision made into the tissue of the perineum. In actual fact, when the baby's head is pressing so hard on the stretching perineal tissue, a natural anesthesia occurs. Your wife would not even feel the incision. However, to the majority of people, the thought of an incision in that delicate area sends them up the walls.

Since the mid-1950s a battle over the episiotomy has been waged between advocates of natural childbirth (not to be confused with prepared childbirth) and obstetricians. Those supporting natural childbirth maintain that the episiotomy is not necessary. But performing an episiotomy is an obstetrical decision. Most physicians who regularly deliver prepared women defer that decision until the time of delivery. They do not routinely perform episiotomies, but use them only when necessary. The considerations that go into the decision are based mostly on the condition of the woman's perineum, its elasticity, and the progress of delivery.

An episiotomy is a prophylactic measure much like your training course has been. It has its place in the prevention of unnecessary trauma. First, if your physician sees at delivery that the perineum is expanding without stretching, it is his judgment based on years of experience and hundreds of deliveries that your wife will tear. He will perform an episiotomy. This will prevent a tear like one in a fabric, jagged and uncontrolled.

Some people say, "Well if I am going to tear, what is the difference between that and an episiotomy?" The answer is an important one. An episiotomy is a small, controlled, straight surgical incision. A tear, or laceration, occurs under tremendous pressure and can involve not only the skin tissue but also much deeper tissue and muscle. This is a complication that should be avoided whenever possible. An episiotomy heals easily; a laceration can lead to problems with elimination after delivery.

A second consideration involves both mother and baby. Prolonged second stage creates a situation in which the baby's head and mother's vagina are in contact under pressure for a long period of time. This can result in long range problems for the mother whose vaginal walls are being weakened by the overly long expulsive effort. Cystocele and/or rectocele, which involve the organs of elimination and their relation to the weakened vaginal wall, can become a real problem to the woman in middle life. These problems are embarrassing at the least and usually require surgical repair so that the woman can completely control her bladder and bowels again.

For the baby, prolonged delivery means unnecessarily long pressure on his head. Even though his head is designed to mold or shape itself to the mother's birth passages, there is no way of judging how an extended second stage may affect the baby's potential for intellectual development.

Based on these factors, no sane parent should object to an

episiotomy, when necessary. It is and it should be a medical decision made at the time of delivery.

Use of forceps

Another form of obstetrical intervention which may occur in the delivery room is the use of forceps. If the doctor feels that the baby is having difficulty being born, he may assist. He does this with forceps, which are instruments that fit along each side of the baby's head and are used to help guide the head around the bony structures inside your wife.

Forceps can be frightening looking. They are made up of two identical sides that cross and can be hinged together. Each side is made of a smooth metal arm on the end of which is a metal elipse. It looks rather like an elongated circle with a hole in the middle. This is the part that fits alongside the baby's head. If the doctor does decide forceps are necessary, your wife will find her breathing techniques helpful. The obstetrician will insert each arm of the forceps separately, guiding it into place with his own hand. This is particularly uncomfortable as the birth area is already distended with the baby and the insertion of equipment does add pressure.

To help your wife relax and cooperate, encourage her to use shallow breathing and concentrate on relaxing the perineum in particular. The insertion of the forceps is accomplished quickly, especially when the woman is able to decrease the resistance by consciously relaxing. Once both arms of the forceps are in place, your obstetrician will attach them at the point outside your wife's body where they overlap. He will then be ready to work with the next contraction. With his permission, your wife can again push, and both will be working together.

It should be mentioned that the use of forceps is just to guide the baby. The doctor will not be pulling him out as many people believe. Therefore, your wife's pushing will be helpful in providing the force, and he can help by providing the direction.

Coaching at moment of birth

Your wife's efforts during delivery are extremely important. As coach, it is your responsibility to see that she is working in concert with the rest of the team. You may find that her concentration during contractions is so intense that she literally blocks out all stimuli. While this is desirable during labor, in the delivery room she needs to be able to respond to the instructions the doctor will be giving her. Since your place is beside her head, it is logical that you should relay the doctor's orders. You can speak directly into her ear and the sound of *your* voice, which has been coaching her efforts throughout labor, can penetrate her concentration. This is especially valuable at the point when the baby's head is about to be born.

As the baby moves down toward the birth outlet, his head is forcing itself against constant resistance. If your wife continues to push effectively, her force will cause the baby to continue to move out at the same rate. One minute he will be resisted by vaginal tissue; the next he will be resisted by nothing but air.

This sudden decompression is not desirable for either mother or baby. And so, as the baby's head is about to be born, the doctor will suddenly say in the midst of a contraction, "Stop pushing." You should repeat this command to your wife and tell her to relax and do her shallow breathing. The uterus will continue to contract, and the obstetrician will manipulate the perineal tissue so that the baby's head can be born gently. By this time, you and your wife will no doubt be straining to see exactly what is going on.

When the contraction subsides, the doctor will be busy with the baby's head. Although it is the only part of the baby outside at this point, the doctor will be preparing the oral and nasal passages for that first breath. He does this by sucking out under gentle pressure the mucus and amniotic fluid that have collected in the baby's nose, mouth, and throat.

The apparatus he uses may be a long thin tube with a glass

bulb attached to the middle, or it may be a bulb similar to an ear syringe. Whatever the particular equipment used, the passages will be cleared so that when the baby takes his first breath, he will not aspirate all that junk into his lungs. Sometimes, if the baby is born faster, this procedure is not done until the baby is completely born. But it is always done before the baby is encouraged to cry.

With the next contraction, the doctor will ask your wife to push to help deliver the shoulders. Once the shoulders are born, there is nothing really obstructing the baby's birth. You may be amazed how quickly the baby is completely born.

APPEARANCE OF THE NEWBORN

Most people are unprepared the first time they see a newborn at birth. All of us have a preconceived notion about the bundle of joy we would like to see. Expecting to see a cute, pink, wriggling, squalling baby, most people are concerned at first sight. No need to be. The majority of infants are exactly as expected within a few minutes of birth. But at the first moment you see him, you can expect the baby to look quite dark. The skin will have a dusky blue quality. This is because, although his body has been receiving adequate nutrients and oxygen, he has not really breathed on his own, and his blood is not nearly as saturated with oxygen as it will be after his first big inspiration.

The second thing you will probably notice is that the baby's skin will have patches of white cheesy material and may be streaked with bright red, mucus-looking blood. The white material is called vernix caseosa. It is a protective coating which serves to protect the baby's skin during its long immersion in amniotic fluid. The bloody streaks can be frightening. It is always upsetting for parents to see blood on their child no matter what his age. But this time there is no need for concern. As the baby moved down the birth canal, he passed many of the surface

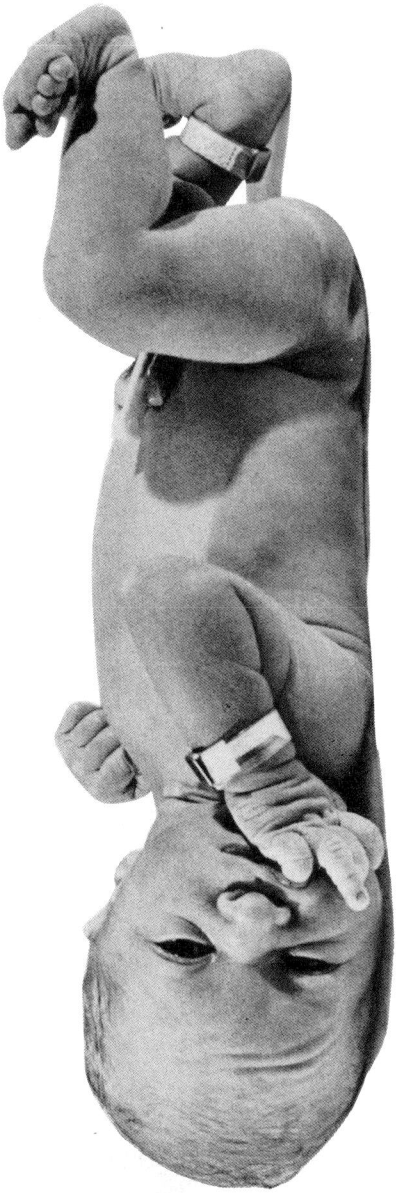

Figure 15. *A HEALTHY NEWBORN BABY: Many parents are unprepared the first time they see a newborn baby at birth.*

capillaries that ooze small amounts of blood during labor. So the streaks that you see on his skin are not his blood at all.

Once the baby is completely born, the doctor will hold him so that his head is down. The force of gravity will help drain off any additional mucus. If he did not have a chance earlier to suction the baby's mouth and nose, the doctor will do so now. Even though the baby is still attached by the umbilical cord to your wife, the doctor will in all probability hold him so that both of you can see him, upside down in all his glory. By this time, most babies have begun to move their arms and legs, and they may be making fussing noises readying themselves for that first big cry which will expand their lungs and set them to breathing on their own.

Stimulating first cry

Some babies do need stimulation. Today a baby is stimulated by stroking his back or flicking the soles of his feet. The old days of whacking the baby on the fanny are gone, as is the tradition of plunging him into water baths. These extreme measures of stimulation have passed into history as more is discovered about the delicate mechanisms of survival within the neonate, or newborn child. For with that first breath, the baby expands his heretofore unused lungs and literally closes the circulatory system that sustained him as he opens the vessels which will support his body for the rest of his life. He is in a whole new world. His body is being called upon to function for itself. All of this happens within a few seconds after birth. You can literally see it going on with your own eyes. While your wife and child are still joined, the baby will open his mouth and utter that most welcomed cry. As he continues to cry, you will actually be able to see pinkness spread over his body.

Your doctor will be quite busy with the baby. At first, he will hold him to facilitate breathing and then, at the proper moment, he will separate him from your wife. For the whole nine months, the baby's life support system has depended on the umbilical cord to carry oxygen and nutrients to his body and waste products away from it. As soon as the baby is breathing on his own, the cord is unnecessary and stops functioning. The physician can tell this has happened because the pulse that could be felt in the cord at birth disappears. When he notes this, the doctor is ready to cut the cord.

This is an absolutely painless procedure for both mother and baby. And, in fact, the mother must be told it is happening or she will not know it. The doctor will put two clamps on the cord about two inches apart. He will then cut between them. In this way, there can be no oozing from either the mother's side or the baby's side. He will then put a more permanent closure on the stump of the cord attached to the baby. Some hospitals have disposable plastic clamps; others still depend on the doctor to tie off the cord by knotting surgical thread around it. It really makes no difference as long as the closure is tight.

As soon as this procedure is completed, the baby will be taken over to the waiting crib. There are a few more things that are done for him, while at the same time the doctor's attention has returned to your wife. So bear in mind that there are really two fields of activity which take place simultaneously.

Identification of baby

Within the first few minutes of life, the baby is provided with identification. When your wife was admitted, a wrist band was prepared for her and two for the baby. The three bands will have the same identification numbers: your wife's hospital number and the band numbers. Most hospitals now use this or a similar system as it is more efficient than the cuter strung name beads of the past. At this time, the baby will have his footprint taken. Some hospitals still use black ink, and you will see traces of it for a few days. Others use an invisible ink that appears when pressed on chemically sensitive paper. On the baby's footprint sheet, the nurse will also imprint one of your wife's fingerprints, usually that of the index finger. In this way, the baby is marked as yours, and you can be sure of proper identification every step of the way.

Also within the first few minutes, the baby's sight is protected. Most states now have laws requiring eye care. In some instances, this means instilling drops and rinsing the eyes. In others it means an injection which provides a systemic protection against infection. This care was instituted in an attempt to control the lifelong problems faced by babies who contract venereal disease at birth.

Mothers sometimes carry organisms in their vagina which do not necessarily cause them any symptoms or problems. However, when the baby passes through that area, he can pick up the organism which is able to flourish in his body and which can cause blindness and other crippling conditions. For this reason, the relatively simple preventive measures were instituted. It should not be looked upon as "dosing" the baby with drugs; it should be seen as an essential part of his perinatal care.

APGAR SCORE

At the first and again at the fifteenth minute of life, the baby is evaluated to see what kind of start he is getting in life. Referred to as the Apgar score, this physical evaluation is sometimes rather unfairly called "the baby's first report card." In parents who need to be competitive, the Apgar score takes on more importance than it really should. They bandy the number around without any real notion of what it measures or how it relates to their own baby.

The Apgar score was developed by Dr. Virginia Apgar, an anesthesiologist, who was trying to evaluate babies' responsiveness. She was particularly concerned with babies whose mothers had been anesthetized.

The evaluation is divided into five points of reference, each assigned a maximum of two points or a minimum of zero points, giving a total of from zero to ten points.

Most normal newborns, who are in excellent health, score from six to eight points. This is based on heart rate, respiratory effort, muscle tone, reflex irritability, and color.

You may see a chart on the wall of the delivery room which will be divided like this:

The Apgar Chart

Sign	0	1	2
Heart Rate	absent	slow (less than 100)	over 100
Respiratory Effort	absent	slow irregular	good crying
Muscle Tone	flaccid	some flexion of extremities	active motion
Reflex Irritability	no response	cry	vigorous cry
Color	blue pale	body pink, extremities blue	completely pink

As you can see, this is not a precise measuring system which can be considered unerringly accurate as a predictor of anything. All it provides is a guideline for evaluating the major areas of response at birth. Its most valuable function is as a point of reference should an infant develop a physical problem during the first few days of life.

It is not a shortcoming if your child scores less than two on any point. For example, most babies score one for color. This is understandable because the baby's circulatory system is just becoming established and his hands and feet are furthest from his heart. In fact, you will probably note for some time that even when the baby is completely pink, his hands and feet will turn blue when he cries. So there is no need for disappointment or elation if you hear a number assigned to your baby. Take him for what he is without attempting to fit him into some category that you might think is suggested by his Apgar score.

When the baby is tagged, printed, and scored, he will be wrapped in a receiving blanket and placed in the crib where he can lie next to the source of oxygen. Some doctors at this point will permit the parents to hold the baby if the business of delivery is complete.

While all of this has been going on with the baby, the doctor and your wife will be working to complete the delivery. Most people believe that once the baby is born, everything is finished. But this is not true. There is yet another piece of business which if not finished can have disastrous consequences. After the baby is born, the organ which provided him with an exchange of oxygen and nutrients for wastes for nine months is no longer needed. The placenta is signalled by an intricate hormone system that it has served its purpose, and it detaches itself from the wall of the uterus.

Removing placenta

What remains at the site of attachment is the mother's side of the story—access to the circulatory system which supplied the placenta. The only way to close this opening is by contracting the uterus and maintaining the muscles contracted. To do this, the placenta must be expelled. Your wife may be asked to push with one or two more contractions after the baby is born. This is the reason. Once the placenta is expelled, the uterus has room to contract down and in most instances will do so spontaneously.

For the woman whose uterus needs an assist at this point, the doctor will order an injection of a hormone to supplement the body's supply. He will also be concerned that all of the placenta has been expelled and will examine the organ. To be positive, most physicians will also do an internal examination. Because of irritability, this examination is uncomfortable. You can remind your wife to do her shallow breathing and relax her perineum as this will help her deal with the sensations and prevent her from tensing and resisting the examination.

The reason that this is so important is that if even a small piece of the placenta is retained, two things can happen. First, it can prevent the uterus from contracting. Then the blood vessels will not be clamped shut, and your wife can have a postpartum hemorrhage. Second, the retained tissue can decompose, releasing waste products that can be poisonous if absorbed into her system. Either complication is best prevented.

Repairing episiotomy

After the placenta is removed, the doctor will add the final touches. This is the time the episiotomy is repaired. You can do your wife a great service if you can divert her attention to the baby. The actual repair is a suturing procedure which is over in a few minutes. However, because of the delicate area in which it is done, this short, relatively painless job can become one of major proportions needlessly. If you can divert her attention, your wife may be aware of annoying pricking sensations during the suturing, but they will be a nuisance, not an issue.

You have completed three stages: labor, delivery of the baby, and delivery of placenta and repair. You and your wife have now arrived at that period called postpartum. You have each done your own job in the business of having your baby. It is an experience to remember the rest of your lives with awe and respect for the miracle of life, and with love and appreciation for each other because of the unique contribution you each have made to the birth experience. You are a family at last.

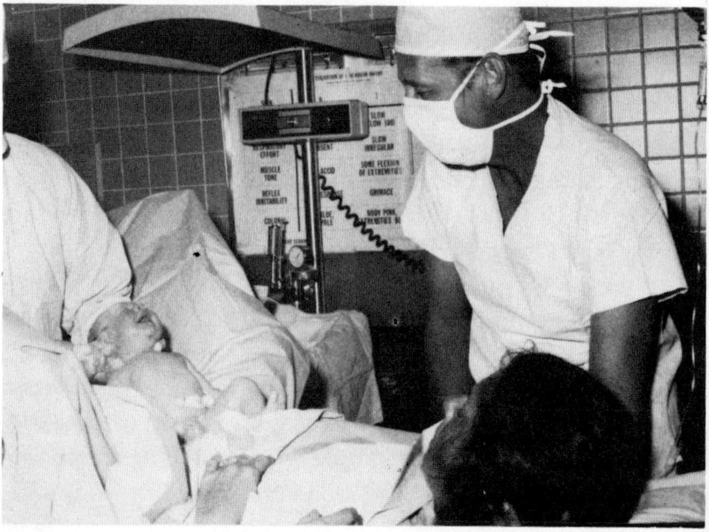

Figure 16. *THE FIRST GLIMPSE: Both parents see their baby for the first time together.*

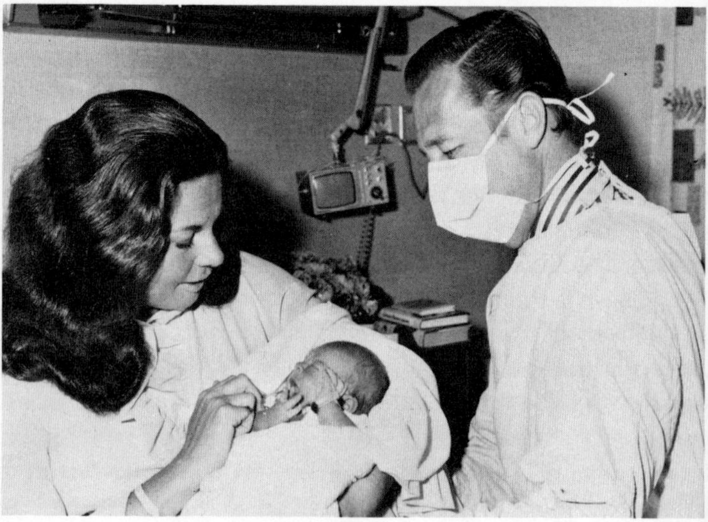

Figure 17. *THE NEW FAMILY: After returning to the hospital room, the parents enjoy a quiet moment with their baby.*

5

In the Hospital Room

Immediately after the baby is born and all of the business of delivery is completed, there will be a time when your wife will be "recovering." This means different things for different women. What hospital people mean by this term is the period until your wife's vital signs—temperature, pulse, and blood pressure—are stable, that is, have returned to normal and are remaining there. Recovery may take place in the delivery room, in which case the delivery table will be returned to its flat condition and your wife will be made as comfortable as possible. Most hospitals today do have a recovery room as part of the labor and delivery suite.

In the recovery room, your wife will be assisted into a hospital bed. During her time in the recovery room, usually a period of one to two hours, a nurse will come in to check a number of things. First, she will verify that your wife's fundus (the upper rounded part of uterus) is remaining firm. Second, she will check the amount of lochia (the discharge of collected blood by the uterus). After birth there is almost always a heavy, bright red flow similar to a heavy menstrual flow. It will decrease in amount and color in the days following birth.

Third, the nurse will ask your wife if she feels the urge to urinate. Although it may seem a strange request considering that your wife has had nothing to drink for several hours, it is possible that urine has collected in the bladder. If the bladder does become full, your wife may not be aware of it because of the various sensations remaining after birth. A distended bladder can force the uterus up out of position and cause it to relax. This does not happen often, but it can be prevented by emptying the bladder. Your wife may find that she can urinate quite easily given the opportunity even though she had not thought of doing so herself.

Perineal control exercises

The recovery period is the ideal time for you to remind your wife to begin her perineal control exercises. By contracting and relaxing the muscles of the perineum at this time, your wife will be preparing her tissues for faster recovery. Still under the influence of the local anesthesia used for the episiotomy, your wife may not think of doing the exercise. Remind her. By doing it now, she will accomplish a few important actions within her body.

First, your wife will improve the muscle tone so that the area will not become "stiff." Most women are afraid to use these muscles after delivery, especially if an episiotomy has been performed. Even though the area does feel sore and there is a tendency to favor it, the exercise is extremely important since the area involves outlets for elimination. By keeping the muscles toned up, your wife will find that she can urinate and defecate without strain or discomfort.

Second, by doing the exercises, your wife will be improving the circulation to an injured area. This is vital in hastening its recovery. Good blood supply provides nutrients and oxygen for repair, and it removes waste products and prevents the collection of fluids which would cause swelling at the site. By instituting these simple exercises during the recovery period, your wife is preparing her body for a quicker recovery so that she can devote her energies to more positive interests, such as preparing for visitors or caring for the baby.

You will probably find that during the recovery period you and your wife both experience a high that is incomparable to any other you have experienced. You have just seen your own baby being born. Together you worked for that moment. And you will relive portions of it for years to come. During the minutes after birth, the two of you will experience a feeling of accomplishment that transcends words.

DELIVERY DAY

As the time slips away, you may both find that your energy is waning despite your good feelings. Do not fight fatigue. Your wife has before your very eyes worked hard to bring your child into the world. Whether she knows it or not, she is physically exhausted. You too are physically and emotionally depleted. Say good-by for a while, tuck her in, and leave. You can rest assured that both she and the baby are well.

Many husbands find that when they finally do leave the hospital and go home, they fall apart. Be prepared for a letdown. You may find that despite the fact that the doctor had the real responsibility for decision-making, you felt a responsibility for your wife and her welfare. You were functioning at a high pitch for most of the active part of labor, during delivery and, of course, after the baby was born. So it is reasonable that as you cool down, your emotions may seem depressed by comparison. It will pass as you are able to get some rest and return to a more normal emotional level. Sleep is as essential for your recovery as it is for your wife's. Plan for a period of sleep, even if it means putting off calling most relatives. Besides, it might be more fun to call them when you and your wife are together again.

During the first twenty-four hours after your wife has delivered, there will be a number of firsts for her and the baby. There will be the first time she gets out of bed. The first time she voids, or urinates. The first time she feeds the baby. The baby too will have his own firsts. The first time he voids. The first time he empties his bowels. The first time he feeds. All of these firsts will be carefully monitored by the hospital staff. It may seem to you an unpleasant preoccupation with basic functions, but they measure a return to normal when they happen or a sign of trouble if they do not.

Your wife may be somewhat troubled the first time she tries to get out of bed. Feeling full of pep and in good spirits flat out in bed, she has no warning of how lightheaded she may become when she puts her feet over the side of the bed for the first time. Her body is responding to the physical exertion of labor and delivery, and it is trying to recover from the sudden changes that occur when the baby is born. Internal pressures change when the baby is no longer inside her body. She has been lying flat or nearly flat for many hours.

Even the force of gravity is against her when she tries to stand up. It will take a few minutes to equalize the blood supply to her brain that occurs just with change of position. Therefore, your wife should be aware that this can occur and wait for a nurse to be with her the first time she tries to get out of bed.

Passing blood clot

There is a good chance that the woman getting up for the first time after delivery will pass a sizable blood clot. This side effect may be somewhat disconcerting to her, but it is logical if you think about the physiology involved. Lying flat in bed causes the vagina to be tipped backwards like a cup. Blood that would normally be discharged as a flow, pools in the vagina and forms a clot. When the woman stands up, the vagina tips forward and pours out the clot.

As long as the uterus is contracted, there is no danger. This is just a sign that the site where the placenta was attached is still oozing. A nurse, and possibly a physician, will probably check to make sure that the fundus is still hard. The incident will be reported to your own doctor, but there is no reason for alarm. Even if the uterus is less firm than the doctor thinks it ought to be, he can show your wife how to gently massage it and/or he will order a dose of hormone, similar to the one used after delivery, to stimulate the uterus to contract.

If your wife has already emptied her bladder in the recovery room, she has proved that her plumbing works. If, for whatever reason, she did not, she will find that the nursing staff will remind her frequently that it is a necessity. It is a good idea for her to drink fluids after delivery—water, juices, coffee, tea—as this will encourage her to produce urine. There are times when the tissue surrounding the urinary openings become edematous, or swollen, during the birth process and it becomes painful or difficult for the woman to void.

Catheterizing

If the woman cannot void after a reasonable amount of time and after consuming a reasonable amount of liquids, the doctor may decide to have the woman catheterized. This is a procedure in which a narrow rubber tube, a catheter, is inserted into the urinary meatus (opening of urethral canal) to provide a pathway for urine to pass out of the body. The edema is not a permanent condition; as soon as it disappears the woman will again be able to urinate without any difficulty. Again, this does not occur commonly. Most women void some time within the first four hours after delivery.

The baby too will be watched closely during the first day of life. Those bodily functions which most of us take for granted are just beginning to become established in the newborn. One of the first bodily functions observed in the newborn is urination. Although he has not taken in any food by mouth, he was nourished by his mother before birth and his body does produce wastes. As he no longer has the convenience of disposing of his wastes through his mother's circulatory system, he will have to get rid of them himself. And so he urinates. This usually occurs some time during the first six hours after birth.

Meconium

The baby may at the same time or shortly thereafter have his first bowel movement. Parents are often disturbed by the color, consistency, and smell if they see it. What the newborn evacuates in his first stool is called meconium. It is largely digested cells, bile, lanugo, and vernix caseosa. It is greenish-black, sticky, and foul smelling but perfectly normal. When the baby starts to feed regularly, the consistency of his stools will change. That meconium movement is just a sign that his bowels are open and ready for action.

Feeding practices differ from culture to culture and from family to family within a given culture. Some people believe that it is imperative to put the baby to breast at the time of delivery. It is true that this does have some advantages, mostly for the mother. The baby's sucking on the breasts stimulates a hormone which encourages the uterus to contract. Also, the baby will receive some colostrum, the only substance in the breast at this time, which provides some nourishment but more importantly stimulates the baby's bowels to function. However, if putting the baby to breast right after delivery is not possible, remember that there is no personal failure involved.

Some pediatricians believe that it is best to allow the baby to rest for the first twelve hours of life. This gives the baby's digestive tract time to begin functioning adequately. They then have the nurse give the first feeding. This is not to deprive the mother of her right to feed the baby. It is purely for safety.

One congenital deformity which can occur without any external signs is called tracheal-esophageal fistula. This is a hole that connects the baby's esophagus with his trachea, or windpipe. If this baby is fed by someone who does not know what to look for, the baby can literally drown in the feeding before there are indications that something is wrong.

This is the reason that the first feeding, usually one of glucose and water, is given to the baby by a nurse. This will in no way interfere with the establishment of breastfeeding provided that the mother does not react in a hysterical way that transmits itself to the baby.

Breastfeeding

Many women who choose prepared childbirth also choose to breastfeed their babies. Many do not. It is neither a feather in the cap of the former nor a cause for distress in the latter. Babies do well with both methods of feeding if the baby is held and mothered at his mealtimes. Breastfeeding advocates tend to overwhelm expectant mothers with the virtues of breastfeeding to the extent that the woman who decides to bottle feed is made to feel that she is less of a mother. This is just not so.

Some women are turned on to breastfeeding and some are definitely turned off. What is important is the relationship between mother and baby when they come together at feeding times. If a mother is most comfortable and relaxed with her baby at breast then this is for her. If she is most comfortable and relaxed bottle feeding her baby then that is *her* choice. What she needs to communicate to her baby is warmth and security. She needs to be able to relax, talk to the baby, cuddle him, and let him know that she is there to take care of him.

To do best by her baby, the mother should make up her mind which method she will use so that she can approach the first feeding ready to master the techniques of that method.

For the expectant mother who wishes to explore the possibilities of breastfeeding, there are a number of books available. Information can also be obtained from La Leche League, headquartered in Franklin Park, Illinois. This organization also provides the names and addresses of mothers around the country who are willing to talk to prospective parents about their successful breastfeeding experiences.

Pediatricians can also supply the desired information. If your wife plans to breastfeed, it is important to choose a pediatrician who favors this method — just as important to your sanity as selecting an obstetrician who believes in prepared childbirth.

The personnel who are responsible for the baby in the hospital are trained to give your wife information about how to put a baby to breast. They will tell her how often and for how long this should be done. However, I wish to add a word of caution.

When your wife starts breastfeeding, the baby is ready but she is not quite set. The baby starts out life with a strong sucking reflex. Even if your wife has been preparing her nipples during the latter part of pregnancy, they still need to be toughened by the actual sucking. For that reason, it is wise for her to begin on a short schedule. She should alternate each side for a few minutes only at each feeding. She can increase the time with each feeding.

In the beginning, the baby will only be getting colostrum as the milk does not "come in" until approximately the third day after birth. As the milk comes in, then, he will be feeding longer to get more. By building up the time, your wife can avoid irritating her nipples. She should get instructions on proper breast care for the nursing mother from her obstetrician. He will tell her what preparations to use to help keep her nipples soft and pliable.

Bottle feeding

For the woman who is intending to bottle feed, there are a number of prepared formulae on the market which attempt to duplicate mother's milk. Discuss this with your pediatrician.

He may have a strong preference based on his experience with infants and their tolerance for the different products. While in the hospital, if your wife is intending to bottle feed, she should be able to attend classes on formula preparation and have her questions answered about vitamin supplements. Most large hospitals now offer this service to mothers who bottle feed their babies.

The baby himself will look somewhat different to you during his first day of life than he did at birth. By the time you see him again, he will be "prettied up." That is, he will have had a sponge bath, been rubbed with baby lotion, and had his hair combed. His general color will be pink, although you may notice that his hands and feet are somewhat dusky. It is interesting to note that all babies are pink in the first day of life even if their parents are dark-skinned. Skin pigment does not develop until later in the life of the infant.

The baby's head may seem big to you. Unlike an adult's, the infant's head is much bigger in relation to his total body. And it is probably not perfectly round. Remember, it had to mold itself to the shape of the birth passages. The baby's head will return to a more normal shape by itself within a few days.

Baby's reflex responses

The baby will sleep almost all of the time unless he is stimulated by one of the visceral influences—hunger, wet, cold, positional discomfort. When he is awake, you will be able to observe the jerky kind of arm flailing, leg writhing movements of the newborn. Awake or asleep, the infant has a number of reflex responses. Sucking, of course, is present. The newborn will suck on any nipple placed in his mouth. If he is hungry and receives nourishment for his efforts, he will continue. If he is not hungry, he will suck for only a few seconds and then go back to sleep.

But before sucking, the infant is equipped with a reflex that is designed to help him find a suitable source of food. Called the rooting reflex, it prompts the baby to turn in the direction of any object that strokes his cheek and to seek a nipple to grasp in his mouth.

The infant also has a strong grasp reflex in both his fingers and his toes. This can be seen when a finger is placed inside the baby's hand; his fingers curl around it and hold it firmly. The same can be done with the toes to the extent that they can curl.

Finally, the infant has a startle reflex sometimes called the Moro reflex. This is seen when the crib is accidentally bumped. The infant will automatically jerk in his arms and legs and duck his head all at the same time. This is a protective mechanism in the tragic instance that a baby might fall. His body forms a ball protecting the important organs and the head. It is a good position for landing.

The presence of these reflexes indicate that the baby's nervous system is functioning. These are the kinds of things, in addition to seeing that all parts are whole, that the pediatrician will look for in that first physical examination which is usually done during the first day.

Full rooming-in

Rooming-in, or having the baby in the same room with his mother instead of in a central nursery, has become more popular with the increased knowledge of early development in infancy. Many new mothers report a sense of deprivation when their infants are taken from their bedside and returned to a central nursery where they can only be seen through a glass wall. By keeping the baby beside her, the new mother is able to watch his antics and learn how to communicate with her own child.

Each baby, like each adult, has his own set of signals. No two babies cry exactly the same way. By having the baby remain at the bedside, the new mother can learn how her own baby cries, and why. This is a simple procedure. When the baby cries, the mother makes a line check. Is he wet? cold? hungry? uncomfortable? bored? If she cannot discover why the baby is crying, sometimes just picking him up and talking soothingly to him will be enough to quiet him and allow him to fall back to sleep. It is far easier for the mother to learn this lesson when she is within call of a nurse than to wait until she is home and completely on her own.

Taking care of the baby in the hospital really should involve more than just feeding him, although for the first day this may be all the mother who has newly delivered has energy to do. There will be a nurse available who is responsible for the care of the infant. During the first day, she should be available to change the diapers as necessary and give the baby his daily sponge bath.

Learning basic care

This is a time for the mother to watch to see how things are done. Most nurses who are accustomed to working with mothers and babies enjoy showing and telling the new mother how to give basic care to the baby. Of course, it is easier for the nurse just to do it! So if your wife has any questions she should speak up. Even though having a baby is a normal part of living, just being in a hospital situation intimidates most people.

Professionals who do an excellent job and do it regularly often forget that new parents do not have the same information or skills at their fingertips. They need to be reminded. Neither you nor your wife should feel at any time that the doctor or nurse will think less of you for asking questions. Just keep telling yourself that somebody had to show them too when they were about to take care of a baby for the first time. With that thought in mind, it is a little easier to ask what you want and need to know.

Many hospitals are not equipped to have a full-time rooming-in situation for all parents. They offer an alternative usually called modified rooming-in which permits the baby to remain at the mother's bedside from early morning through most of the day until afternoon visiting hours.

'Father's hour'

In this situation, the hospital usually provides for a "father's hour." For some institutions this is during the early evening so that the father may be present during the baby's evening meal. In other institutions, this may be an extension of the evening visiting hours in which all other visitors are excluded and the father may visit with mother and baby. So whether there is full rooming-in or modified rooming-in, most hospitals that call themselves family-centered now do make a provision for the father to be with and handle his child in those days directly after birth.

The first day after birth is really a day of getting to know. You and your wife will be getting to know your baby. You will be getting to know what is expected of you during your wife's stay. It is a time of adjusting. Do not expect miracles. *There is no such thing as instant motherhood or fatherhood.* You will be the same person the day of delivery that you were the day before. You will have the same feelings and maybe even some of the same doubts that you had before the baby was born. The only thing that has changed in your lives is that the baby is here. You have to learn how to be parents just as you learn any other roles. It is a growing relationship between you and the baby, you and your wife, and your wife and the baby. The three of you are a unit.

Fear of being left out

Most fathers are afraid that once a baby is born they will be replaced in their wife's affection. This is a normal reaction. However, if the father sees his family as one composed of members who are equal in importance and stature, he does not need to feel left out. Being with and handling the baby in the hospital help many fathers to overcome the feeling of being left out.

Taking part in the baby's care later at home will do even more to enhance the unity of the family.

POSTPARTUM ONE

The second day after delivery is called postpartum day one. By now your wife is beginning to return to her usual interest in her own appearance in addition to her acute interest in the baby. The doctor will probably allow her to take a shower if all has gone well up to this point. Baths are taboo and will remain so until the uterus has returned to its preconception state several weeks after delivery. This is because the cervix is still open and the placental site is a direct pathway to her blood stream. A minor vaginal infection at this stage of the game could easily be spread throughout the body leading to a life-threatening septicemia. Well worth avoiding.

You will be surprised how being able to shampoo her hair will make your wife feel like a human being again. But you will not be so pleased by her reaction to her shape. For some reason, most people think that once the baby is born, the new mother is going to be able to model for fashion magazines. Well, this just is not so. It took nine months for her figure to achieve its predelivery shape. It will take several weeks for it to return to what it was before she was pregnant.

Postpartum exercises

Most women are dismayed when they see themselves for the first time after delivery and discover that they still look a little pregnant—about five month's worth. Those abdominal muscles just need to firm up. There are two simple, nonstrenuous exercises which can be done in the hospital which are designed to firm up a flabby belly. But, as with any exercises, they *should not* be started until the doctor has given his permission. This is extremely important as most doctors have their own ideas about just what exercises should be begun on what day postpartum.

The first exercise is called a head lift. It is done lying on the back. A pillow may be placed under the knees. As with any exercise, it is begun with a deep breath, in and out. After the second deep inhalation, the head is raised slowly until the chin touches the chest as the breath is exhaled. With the third inhalation, the head is slowly lowered to the bed again. This exercise may be done five times twice a day while your wife is in the hospital.

The second exercise is called abdominal isometrics. It should be done standing preferably although it can really be done in any position. It is begun with a deep inhalation-exhalation. As the next breath is inhaled, the abdominal muscles are contracted until they cannot be contracted any further. The idea is to attempt to reach the spine by pulling in the belly. These muscles are held for a slow count of five. The muscles are slowly released as air is exhaled. This exercise should be done five times, twice a day while in the hospital.

Chosen specifically for postpartum recovery by registered physical therapist Polly De Santo, these exercises will strengthen the abdominal muscles and help your wife to return to her former shape, if that is her goal. You might try them yourself if you are beginning to develop a paunch. Our routine activities do not encourage men or women to use the abdominal muscles with any regularity. These two exercises can help you both get into a shape you would be proud to put into a bathing suit. You might consider making them a permanent addition to your regular exercise pattern.

Feeling more like herself, your wife may be ready to participate more in the baby's care by this day. For some reason, many women who are very capable of caring for young children suddenly forget their skills when they are presented with a child of their own. So do not be surprised if your normally confident wife seems to lack her usual self-assurance. This is just a reaction to motherhood and its terrifying responsibilities. Once given the opportunity to sharpen her skills under the guidance of a nurse in the hospital, your wife will be able to take over and do a great job. But she will need all of your support for those first struggling attempts.

The only real stumbling block that might be unforeseen in the care of the newborn is his bath. For until the baby's cord has dried and fallen off (and it will by itself), bathing means a sponge bath. This is a simple procedure which takes about five minutes.

Changing diapers

Sometimes professionals create such a mystique around simple maneuvers that the ritual becomes more important than the job being done. Do not let your wife become so concerned about doing things right that she does not do them at all. Encourage her to do things for the baby. Changing diapers may not be her idea of a fun job, but unless she has someone who will do it for her at home, it is better for her to get the hang of it while she can still ask questions than to wait until you bring them home and then have to turn to the pediatrician.

There are a great many things to learn about changing the baby that will all come automatically after a while. Primarily the most important thing to learn is what the baby looks like and should look like. This may sound funny but it is not. How many new parents are prepared for the size and shape of the genitals of a newborn? They are considerably larger in proportion than in the adult. Did you know that newborn girls may have a vaginal discharge similar to a mini-menstrual discharge? If your wife never takes the diaper off the baby in the hospital, she may not see this until you are home. Then panic sets in.

In addition to the way that the baby looks normally, it is important for your wife to know how to recognize and deal with rashes that might occur. "Red bottom" can occur for a number of reasons—irritating urine, detergent in the diaper—and may occur within the first few days. It is treated ideally by keeping the baby's bottom dry. This can be done by applying moisture proof products after cleansing the area. It can be done by leaving the diaper off and placing the baby on his belly to sleep. All of these things can be learned in the sheltered situation of the hospital if your wife is willing to use the time as one to discover her own abilities by caring for the baby.

This is not an attempt to ease the work for the nurses. It is far easier to do it quickly and be done than it is to help someone less sure to do the job and learn from it. You, too, can use your time with the baby to learn about his care. While most fathers are not available to care for a baby at all times, many do want to pitch in when they can. Let your wife show you what she has learned. It will help her to be able to show you, and then if the two of you have any questions, the nurse is not far away.

Baby's sponge bath

In daily routine, the baby's sponge bath should be accomplished with as little excitement as possible. When the baby gets somewhat older, the bath will be the high point of his day. But for the first few weeks, the bath is just to make him clean and comfortable.

There is nothing dramatically different about sponging a baby. You should start at his head and work down. Before putting any soap in the water use clean, moistened cotton balls to wipe the baby's eyes. Using a separate cotton ball for each eye, wipe gently going from the inner to the outer corner. Then discard the cotton ball. The explanation is simple. You do not want to get soap into his eyes; that is why you do it first. Soap will irritate him as much as it would you, and he does not have functioning tear ducts yet to wash out his eyes as you would.

After you cleanse the eyes, your next target is the baby's head. Lying in a crib, the baby will tend to collect stale food and other particles in his hair. If these are allowed to build up, a condition known as cradle cap will develop. This can be prevented by shampooing the baby's head.

This is also a simple deal. By supporting the baby's back on your forearm and keeping his body between your arm and hip, you can effectively hold the baby so that he cannot wiggle, and you still have a free hand for his care. In this position, his head will rest in the palm of your hand. It is a perfect position for shampooing, sometimes called the football hold. Holding him this way, cup some water from the bath in your hand and moisten his head. Work a small amount of soap into a lather and apply it to the baby's scalp.

Soft spots, or fontanels

Do not be afraid to touch the baby's head. Even though the bones do not meet, and there are soft spots called fontanels, the baby's brain is protected and you cannot hurt it by manipulating his scalp. The presence of the fontanels allowed the baby's head to mold to the birth canal and will allow for continued brain growth. They will not close until the child is around the age of one. So you might as well get used to them. After you have lathered, rinse the baby's scalp by cupping water. Then towel dry.

The rest of the bath is a snap. Moisten the baby down his front side. Lather sparingly, being sure to clean out all of the creases as these hidden places are where food and dirt collect and cause irritation. Rinse him off and towel. Turn him over and do the same for his back side. When he is clean and dry you can apply a baby lotion of your choice. Use it sparingly, too. A quarter-size dab rubbed between your hands and run over the baby's skin will make him smell nice. Too much can clog his pores and cause him to run a fever.

The last step is to dress him and then hold him and talk to him and make him feel that his life will not always be such a turmoil. Once clean and dry and secure, the baby is ready for his next meal.

POSTPARTUM TWO

The third twenty-four hour period after delivery, or P.P.2, may be more traumatic for your wife than any preceding day. In that period, forty-eight to seventy-two hours after birth, the baby will go through a subtle change. His skin will develop a yellowish caste. And the sclera (white area) of his eyes may even become yellow-tinged. Being well-prepared for motherhood, your wife will undoubtedly have read everything she could get her hands on relative to the baby and how he will develop. This includes, of course, all the things that can go wrong.

In today's literature, there has been a great deal of publicity about the advances being made in the treatment of blood incompatabilities. Anyone who has read these articles knows that jaundice, or yellowing of skin, is a sign that the baby's blood is incompatible with his mother's and that her antibodies transmitted to the baby are destroying his red blood cells. What is not clear is that this condition, technically named erythroblastosis fetalis, produces its symptoms during the *first* twenty-four hours of life.

The baby who begins to become jaundiced during his third day is demonstrating icterus neonatorum, or physiological jaundice. It occurs because the baby's immature liver is not yet able to handle the increased load of blood pigment produced when his body attempts to eliminate extra red blood cells. There is no specific treatment, although some pediatricians have found that sunlight seems to help reduce the jaundice. The condition usually clears up by itself within one to two weeks. It is mentioned here because during the P.P.2 day, your wife is especially vulnerable and needs your support. She may notice the baby's change in color and her reaction may be very emotional. You can help to calm her if you know about physiological jaundice.

Rest assured, if there are any real problems with the baby, the doctors will tell you as soon as a diagnosis has been made. You are the baby's parents. Your permission must be given before any treatment, save emergency first aid, can be given to your baby. But your wife has cause to be emotionally brittle at this time.

During the days after delivery, the highly complex hormonal signalling system struggles to establish a new pattern within your wife's body. First, the hormones of pregnancy are no longer necessary. Second, the hormones that return your wife to her prepregnant state are working overtime, and third, the hormones which produce nourishment for the just-delivered baby are hard at work and yielding significant results between the second and third day after delivery.

These complex internal changes can play havoc with your wife's emotions. One minute she is happy and elated about your beautiful new baby. The next she is in tears about something as trivial as a menu change on her luncheon tray. For nine long months she has been the center of the universe. All her goals were directed toward the baby. She worked and practiced with you, and her efforts reached a climax with the baby's birth. And then what? Everybody from her mother to her best friend comes to see the baby. She feels like she has been forgotten.

You may be feeling some of this too, but your hormones are not adding insult to injury. So, it is up to you to try to restore some of your good feelings together. This is a good time to give your wife a gift—something especially for her, having nothing to do with the baby. If you are planning to celebrate, bring a split of champagne for the two of you to toast each other. Third days are hard for new mamas. But you can make it easier by showing your wife that she is still important to you. After you have done that, then both of you together will be able to enjoy the baby.

This emotional letdown experienced by most women about the third day is called baby blues or postpartum blues. It is expected. It is normal. If pampered, most women can be easily restored to feeling good. If the letdown is ignored, it can often grow out of proportion with the new mother unconsciously seeking attention in other ways. So it is well worth your effort to remember that your wife worked darned hard and to give her the credit and attention that is due her.

Values of colostrum

As mentioned before, about this time, your wife's milk is coming in. This may sound strange since you may have noticed a yellowish white liquid secreted from her breasts since before the baby was born. What you saw was a substance called colostrum. It is somewhat different from the breast milk that your wife will produce in that it is higher in protein, lower in fat and carbohydrate. But it has two properties that make it valuable to the baby. First, it is a natural laxative. And second, it contains some antibodies which may play an important part in enhancing the immunity of the newborn.

When the baby suckles during the first few days, he is receiving colostrum. His sucking action serves to stimulate the production of milk, also known as lactation. This process will occur to some extent even in the woman who is not stimulated by the baby's sucking. But her supply of milk will gradually diminish. When the milk does come in, the initial reaction within the breast is as if the tissue had been invaded by a foreign protein. For a day or so, the breasts will be full, hard, and tender. This is a difficult time for new mothers. The baby may have trouble grasping the nipple because of the hardness of the surrounding breast tissue. This will add to your wife's emotional reactions.

It is a time when she will need a great deal of encouragement. If you both felt strongly in favor of breastfeeding before the birth, it is worth persisting during this difficult period. By continuing to nurse and encouraging the milk to flow, the engorgement will disappear. But it does take perseverance and support.

For the woman who is not breastfeeding, engorgement will also occur unless medication has been given to inhibit lactation. For her, the act of not putting the baby to breast will eventually cause the breasts to dry up from lack of stimulation. Some women given medication at delivery to forestall lactation find that they experience a delayed lactation which appears about ten days to two weeks after delivery.

If your wife is planning to bottle feed, you should discuss with your obstetrician whether or not he should administer any medication that will interfere with lactation. Your wife might fare better by allowing lactation and the resulting engorgement to occur in the sheltered environment of the hospital where someone can offer her comfort measures and completely take over the care of the baby if necessary.

POSTPARTUM THREE

Many physicians are now sending mother and baby home on the third day postpartum. In some hospitals, the stay is even shorter. This trend toward shorter hospitalization for normal labor, delivery, and postpartum is a result of the recognition of the normalcy of the process. Once certain that mother and baby are free from postpartum complications, the physicians are willing to allow them to return home to begin functioning as a family in a natural setting.

There are other factors that have led to this development. One is the threat of many young couples to have home deliveries. Considered unsafe by most obstetricians, who prefer to have the latest equipment and highest trained personnel at hand in case of emergency, home deliveries gained popularity among couples who refused to be separated for the birth of their child. As a compromise, many physicians allow the couple to stay home during most of labor, deliver at the hospital, and return home as soon as medically feasible for mother and baby after birth. In this way, both mother and baby can be offered optimal safety and the family can still be together for the birth.

Another factor that has pressured doctors to release healthy mothers and babies earlier is the spiralling costs of hospitalization. This is of special concern to the majority of families who are not yet financially established. In many areas of the United States, the cost of having a baby—the obstetrician's fee and the hospital—runs between $600 and $1,000. Therefore, in an attempt to reduce needless cost to young families, physicians are willing to discharge on the third day postpartum.

When you come to take your family home, you will need to bring clothes for your wife and for the baby. Your wife may have laid them out before you took her to the hospital in labor. But it is a good idea if you check them anyway, just in case she forgot something.

Many parents bring the most adorable sets of clothing for dressing the baby to go home. Even though well intentioned, this is patently ridiculous. There is no reason on earth why a four-day-old infant has to wear underwear, a starched dandy suit, and a woolen blanket set in the middle of July. In the first place, all clothes to go on the baby should be soft and loose fitting. He needs room to move and kick inside his wrappings. In the second place, the infant responds to the weather much the same way as you do. If it is too hot for you to wear an overcoat, it is too hot for him to have four layers of clothing. Use common sense in dressing the baby. Do not forget that in an air conditioned nursery, where the temperature is kept at a constant cool, the baby was dressed only in a diaper, an undershirt, and a cotton receiving blanket. Take this as a cue.

Most hospitals have similar routines for discharging mother and baby. It is usually after the morning feeding for the baby and

For your wife, you will need:

a dress—loose fitting is essential—if she does not have this kind of dress in her wardrobe, bring along one of her dressier maternity dresses.

a slip

panties—cotton is preferable

brassiere—maternity or good supporting

girdle—if she normally wears one and has doctor's permission

pantyhose—many are now available in one size that fits all, and are easier to manage than stockings and a girdle

shoes—comfortable ones that blend esthetically with the dress you are bringing

coat or sweater—depending on the weather and on what your wife already has with her at the hospital.

For the baby, you will need:

two diapers—at least

two undershirts—in case one is soiled, you will have a change

one camisole

one blanket set—the number of pieces and weight of this set should be determined by the weather.

before the lunchtime for the mother. The first step is also usually the same—you make arrangements to pay the bill. The billing department will give you some kind of receipt which you bring up to the floor on which your family has been staying.

When you present the receipt to the floor nurse, she will send someone to help you dress the baby. Actually you and your wife are perfectly capable of dressing the baby, but the final details of identification must be verified. Your wife will probably be asked to verify the footprint and fingerprint taken in the delivery room and to sign the same sheet attesting to the identification for the record.

A member of the nursing staff will accompany you down to the street where you will have your car waiting. For safety reasons, she will carry the baby, placing him on your wife's lap once she is seated in the car. If you are planning to travel by public transportation, it might be wise if you invested in a taxicab as you will have the luggage, the baby, and your wife, all needing your attention.

The day does come when you and your wife and your baby are on your way. You are taking your family home.

6

After Returning Home

You may find that your feelings as you ride home with your wife and child for the first time are somewhat mixed. Although happy to have them with you as you drive away from the protective atmosphere of the hospital, you may begin to feel the awesome sense of responsibility that sometimes accompanies being a new parent. Your wife undoubtedly will have many of the same feelings. After all, until now there has always been someone nearby to help make decisions about the baby. Now you are on your own.

Do not let your feelings overwhelm you. Talk about them with your wife. She will be glad to know that she is not alone in her insecurity. Once out in the open, your fears can be reduced to manageable levels. You and your wife *are* capable of being good parents. You really will know what to do. It is not that you are sure that you will do something wrong, an unlikely possibility. It is truly that you are afraid of the unknown. This is a very human reaction. You can prepare yourself to take care of your baby just as you prepared yourself to work with your wife to deliver him.

Many people plan well in advance of birth to have a baby

nurse come home with them to take care of the baby. *This is a cop out.* It is true that your wife will not have all the energy she needs to take care of herself, the baby, and the house. What she needs is to have someone help her do the daily things that need to be done—cooking and cleaning. She certainly does not need someone who will do the thing that she needs to learn and can learn best by practice—how to care for her baby. The most important thing that your wife has to do when she gets home is to take care of herself and to take charge of the baby.

The baby, too, needs to be taken care of by his mother. More and more, psychologists are discovering that the first few weeks after birth have a significant role to play in the emotional development of the child. It is important for the baby to get to know the most important people in his life, his mother and his father. He learns this by the way he is answered when he cries.

Crying is the only way the young infant has of communicating. He cries whenever he is uncomfortable; he does not differentiate whether his discomfort is physical or emotional. When he cries, it should be one of his parents who goes to him, tries to find what is troubling him, and moves to correct it. By paying attention to his cries, you are teaching him that there is something outside of himself. Contrary to common belief, you do not spoil a small infant by attending his cries. In fact, you are giving him a better start in life if he learns that he can trust his parents to take care of his needs. This is something that you can do better than any hired professional, no matter how warm and loving she may seem.

You and your wife will learn quickly to differentiate between the baby's cries for food, for a diaper change, or for company. If you can teach the baby that you are there to answer his cries early in the game, you will find that you have an easier time with him as he gets older. For if the baby knows that you are there, he can begin to learn to wait. He will trust you to come to him as soon as you are able. It is a two-way street. The baby communicates his feeling of trust to you. When you are communicating with each other, parent to child and child to parent, then you truly have a family.

Providing housekeeping help

Saying that your wife should be caring for the baby is not to minimize her depleted energies. It will take several weeks for her to return to her normal energy level. She will definitely need help to keep a house running. If it is at all possible, the best arrangement is for you to plan to take your vacation from the day of the baby's birth. If your wife is a fussy housekeeper, you should get the house in order before you bring her home. If she can live with a little disorder, so much the better for you. But by being available twenty-four hours a day, you are continuing the same kind of emotional support that you gave her during labor.

This is essential for any woman after delivery. Not only is she physically exhausted, she is mentally and emotionally drained. She desperately needs someone who can baby her while she begins to take on the responsibility of caring for the baby. As her husband, you can do this job best. And there is a definite advantage in it for you. You will be at home and able to observe and participate in the care of the baby. You are really starting out a new life together. You can help each other by being together. Your teamwork made labor an experience to remember. Being parents should further your abilities to function as a unit, a family.

If it is not possible for you to take a vacation at the time of the baby's birth, it would be well worth the expense of having someone come in to help with the household chores. It is not necessary to have anyone live in. In fact, it is advisable for you to spend your free time alone with your family to get to know them and see yourself in your new role as father.

Unless your wife has a particularly good relationship with

either her mother or your mother, the grandmothers should not be encouraged to move in "for a couple of weeks." Usually friction develops between the generations, no matter how well-meaning the intentions. Discord is the last thing that you want in your household when there are so many variables that depend on smooth communication. This is not to say the grandparents should not visit. On the contrary, they have a right to see the baby. But they must understand that their presence is desired in limited quantities so as not to further drain your wife's already depleted resources.

Limiting visitors

Visitors in general should be limited if possible. Well-meaning friends and relatives will undoubtedly telephone and try to visit from the time the baby is in the hospital. If you are home, you should make it a practice to screen calls. Long conversations may be unnecessarily tiring for your wife. Find out who is calling and whether or not she wants to take the call. If she does, remind her to keep it short. As during your wife's pregnancy, you will be serving as a kind of watchdog *but not a bully*. Point out what is best. But she is a big girl and should be allowed to make up her own mind. Just remind her.

Personal visitors are a little more difficult to discourage. It is not a particularly good idea to have many different people visiting. For while the baby does have some immunities against major diseases to which your wife is immune, he is not any more immune to the common cold than she.

A cold is a disaster when a baby contracts it. Not only is there concern that it will develop into something more serious, but the baby will have difficulty with just the simple activities of living. Young babies are not mouth breathers, and trying to breathe through blocked nasal passages is hell. It is almost impossible for the baby to suck since he cannot coordinate his usual sucking-breathing pattern. Short Eustachian tubes provide direct passage of infection to the inner ears leading to painful swelling. Is it not simpler to avoid a cold by limiting visitors?

One way some couples have gotten around the visiting problem is to schedule a welcoming party when the baby is about one month to six weeks of age. Visitors with colds are still excluded, but at least such a party gives your wife a chance to get back on her feet so that she can enjoy her guests. And friends and relatives do not feel so put out if their request to visit is not just turned down but countered with an invitation.

Avoiding jealousy

The question raised by most new parents, whether this is their first baby or not, is how do we avoid the problem of jealousy when we bring the baby home? For parents with other children, it is of course the older child for whom they are concerned. For first-time parents, it is usually a pet, a dog or a cat, who until the baby was born enjoyed the spotlight, being treated as the "baby" of the family. This is a real concern since in either case the baby's physical welfare might be at stake. The answer to the question is one which each couple will have to work out for themselves in the practical sense, but the situation can be explained in a general way. It is important that pets and older children be made to feel that they are just as important as ever in their own right, and that you, the parents, see them as equally important as the baby.

One way this is handled by some couples is to begin this reassurance from the moment mother and baby are brought home. For example, on entering the house, the father will carry the newborn and the mother bring a gift. This allows mother who has been absent from the home, to be warmly greeted without placing the baby as an obstacle to reaching her.

With young toddlers, this is extremely important. Toddlers are especially threatened by separation from mother. By returning home and physically greeting the toddler with affection and enthusiasm, his mother is telling him that he is still very important to her. This established, he can turn his attention to the baby.

With pets, the situation is not altogether different. Pets have a strong proprietary sense about their domain. Bringing a new person into the animal's home requires a time of adjustment so that the pet can become accustomed to the sight, smell, and noises of the baby. It is not a bad idea to bring an edible plaything for the pet.

The gift to be brought home for a pet serves only as a plaything, a distraction. But the gift suggested for the toddler whether boy or girl, is more. The wise parent will be trying to help the toddler to feel a part of the new family. For this reason, the toddler's gift should be a baby doll, one without the frills. This doll provides the toddler with a baby of his own to which he can relate. Identified with the live baby, the doll takes on the baby's attributes and the baby's needs for the toddler. For example, when mother feeds the baby, the toddler feeds the doll. When mother changes the baby, the toddler changes the doll. And it is often observed that when the toddler feels hurt or rejected, it is the doll that receives the toddler's scolding or spanking. This is a healthy way for the toddler to express his feelings. By doing so, the toddler can continue to develop his own mental health without endangering the physical welfare of the baby.

If you cringed during the last paragraph, you have lots of company. The majority of men in our culture think that dolls are just fine for their daughters but that their sons have to learn how to be little men. They believe that the little boy who plays with dolls is a sissy and destined to be effeminate. This is a prejudice based on sexism, not fact. Little boys have just as strong a need to be tender and loving as do little girls. But by denying them the opportunity, parents who want their sons to be little men are often setting up road blocks to the boys' healthy emotional adjustment and to their ability to effectively relate to men and women as an adult.

It is important for little boys, especially when they are toddlers, to have an object upon which they can take out their feelings, both bad and good. Boys learn how to be men by watching and imitating their fathers. Since you intend to hold and play with the baby, you had better find a way for your son to copy your actions.

By providing an asexual baby doll—neither boy nor girl without any of the frills you might give to a little girl—you allow the toddler to participate in the baby's care in a way that is meaningful for him and safe for the baby. And you will find that as the newness wears off, so does the toddler's interest. When the toddler tires of caring for the doll, other things in his world will again be of interest; he will return to the doll only in times of stress when the baby seems a threat to his safe world with Mommy and Daddy.

Period of adjustment

Bringing the baby home can also be an event that disrupts the baby. Be it the change of environment or a general increase in nervous tension in his parents, the baby will go through a period of adjustment too. He may seem fussier to you at home than he was in the hospital. Your wife may point out that he is not feeding on the same schedule. These variations in behavior should be expected and are not cause for alarm. In fact, the calmer you and your wife remain, the sooner you will find that the baby assumes a regular pattern of eating and sleeping. It is your calmness which communicates itself to the baby that helps him feel secure.

Facts about feeding

Eating is a big thing in our society. It is not only food consumption but a social event and a gesture of love. There are so many social and emotional associations that go along with eating that the actual function is of minimal importance. As it is with adults, eating is an important time for the infant. It is a time of warmth, security, and close physical contact with another human being. These factors are just as important to the infant as the milk he ingests. This is why calmness is so strongly emphasized.

Fed by a person who cuddles, talks softly, and handles him with assurance, the baby who eats small amounts frequently is more likely to assimilate what he takes in. Good vibrations help the baby maintain a feeling of security. On the other hand, if the baby is forced to consume a given amount at a given time by a nervous individual who needs to have the baby "eat," the baby is likely to develop problems with digestion such as gas which he cannot expel unaided. The trapped gas causes him pain; he cries and makes his mother more nervous, and a cycle begins. Bad vibrations set the baby up for a pattern of development that is neither physically satisfying nor emotionally healthy.

You can avoid this pitfall by helping to create a calm, quiet environment during the baby's feeding time. As a matter of fact, you can do a great deal during the baby's mealtime. If your wife has chosen to bottle feed the baby, there is no reason in the world why you cannot offer to give the baby his bottle. And if she has chosen to breastfeed, that does not necessarily mean that you need to be totally left out.

Most babies will wake up hungry and in need of a change of diapers. Not only would you be serving yourself with an opportunity to handle the baby, but you would be performing a service for your wife if you took the initiative and offered to bring the baby to her. This will conserve her energy, and you will not be left out just because she has the equipment built in.

Starting a home schedule

Many couples find, especially in the early days of parenthood, that they enjoy caring for the baby together. This does not mean that they are standing on top of each other every moment.

It means that they share the responsibility, helping one another to carry out the daily activities. As time goes on and the husbands can no longer be home all day every day with their families, many couples work out a schedule which permits the father to continue to participate in the baby's care.

In the hospital, the major part of the baby's care is given in the morning. This is usually done because most hospitals are staffed better during the daytime. Upon coming home, many couples fall into the same routine as they observed in the hospital. This is understandable. Being new parents, they want to do everything right. And the hospital is really the only model they have at this time in the care of the baby. But in point of fact, the baby does not have any concept of night and day. He only knows comfort and discomfort.

Therefore, there is no reason in the world why you should continue on the hospital schedule if it deprives you of the chance to see, be with, and care for your child. An arrangement that works out well for many new parents is to postpone the baby's bath until just before the late evening feeding. This gives Daddy time to get home, clean up, and relax. It gives Mommy a feeling that she has not bitten off more than she can chew and that you are there to help her with some of the work. And it gives baby an interesting advantage too that benefits the three of you.

The most prolonged time of comfort for the baby is usually after his bath and the feeding that follows. He is relaxed, sleepy, and comfortable. He usually sleeps longest after that combination of care. Think how you yourself feel after a bath and a good meal. You are ready for a nap too. Well, if this is provided for the baby in the late evening, it is logical that he will be ready for a long sleep. You too will be able to sleep longer. This does not mean that he will not wake for his middle-of-the-night feeding. It does mean that he will probably sleep longer until he wakes.

As most people find that waking in the middle of the night is the most disconcerting part of caring for the newborn, assisting the baby to sleep longer into the night is often a help to them. For some reason, confirmed by experiments, the quality and length of sleep in the early part of the night seem to provide the most refreshment. Therefore making the baby comfortable to sleep an extra half-hour or hour is of some benefit to you as well.

Making check-up appointments

In thinking ahead in the care of your wife and the baby, you should try to remember to have your wife call to make an appointment with both the obstetrician and the pediatrician shortly after you bring her home from the hospital. Your wife will be expected to make a six-week-check-up visit to the obstetrician, and the baby will be seen by the pediatrician some time between the third and fourth week for a routine check up. Both of these visits are precautionary, just to make sure that everything is progressing as expected. The reason for calling so promptly is that if the appointments are not made, often time passes and they are forgotten.

It is important for your wife to know that involution, the returning of the uterus to its prepregnant place, is complete. This should also be of interest to you as theoretically you and your wife are expected to abstain from sexual intercourse until this check up. There are two excellent reasons for this precaution. First, while the cervix is still open, intercourse can introduce infection into the uterus. Organisms that might be found in other parts of the body without causing disease and would ordinarily be destroyed in the vagina, can travel up into the uterus and cause serious complications. Second, although your wife will probably not menstruate during the period after birth, she may well ovulate.

Even breastfeeding mothers may ovulate without menstrual flow during this time. This is mentioned because often advocates of breastfeeding claim family planning as one of the advantages.

While lactation does suppress menstruation, it does not suppress ovulation.

You may say: "So what? We had such a good experience I do not mind having another baby." The answer to that is you should mind for your wife's and child's sake. It takes several months for your wife's body to return to a state where it can accept another pregnancy without tremendous strain on her physical and emotional resources. It is also a disservice to your child to allow your wife to become distracted by another pregnancy before she has even had a chance to get to know this baby.

This does not mean that you should not plan to have another child. It means only that you should plan to have one when it is reasonable for all members of your family.

Sexual tensions during this time can be a problem for both you and your wife. You should not ignore each other just because intercourse is proscribed. As during pregnancy, seek other ways to express your love for each other. You can be tender and physical. And mutual fondling can bring either of you to an orgasm which will help to relieve some of the tensions.

As with almost all other parts of post-pregnancy activities, the resumption of intercourse should be discussed with your obstetrician. It is usually difficult for most people to ask the questions about sex and pregnancy that they want to because of the learned attitudes about sex, even in our liberated society today. But try to remember, the obstetrician is aware that this is one of your concerns. The question can be raised at the time late in pregnancy when he advises you to refrain from intercourse. This is a logical time to ask for how long. You and your wife do not need to be embarrassed about having normal sexual feelings toward each other. Was that not the way the baby came about, after all?

The first visit to the pediatrician is usually a happy event. He will give you a progress report on the baby. Up until that time, you and your wife will probably not be sure that the way you have been caring for the baby has been the right way. At the first visit, you are usually told that the baby has shown growth and development. Each infant develops at a different rate, even in the same family. Therefore there will be no prediction here of exactly what the doctor will say.

But you can be pretty sure that the scale will show that the baby has regained the weight he lost in the first few days and then added some to that. You may be told that he has grown a fraction of an inch. No matter what progress, it will at least give you the feeling that you are doing something right. This will help very much in carrying on with the activities.

Guidelines for good parenting

There should be no hard and fast rules for care of a newborn. Parents for the most part are the best authorities on their own children. This is an idea that new parents find hard to accept. But it is true. For while they are very concerned about doing the physical things for the baby in a correct manner, it is often the intangibles which they do that are so much more important. Therefore, there should be only two guidelines for new parents which if observed will provide a basis for all that follows.

Follow your own instincts. You are reacting to the baby on a basic level when you instinctively try to do something for him. Your warmth and concern for his well-being are communicated. Instincts, after all, educators tell us, are really intellectual short cuts between knowledges that we have and may not even be aware of. There is little you can do to hurt the baby outside of deliberate physical violence. So do try to implement your own ideas. It does not take an expert to learn how to pin on a diaper. It only takes practice. If you pin on enough loose ones which you have to replace, you will learn how to attach it in a better way.

Answer the baby each time he calls. Crying is the only way the baby has of telling you he needs something. By coming to him each time he calls you, you are teaching him his first and most important lesson: there is someone outside of himself on whom he can depend. You cannot spoil a newborn. If you try to make him comfortable each time he lets you know he is in distress, he learns very rapidly that there is warmth and security outside of himself. He learns also that since he can depend on someone outside of himself, he can wait for relief. Not only will you be helping the baby on the first steps to mental health, you will be doing yourself a favor as well. For while you may find that you make many trips to the bassinet in the beginning, the frequency of his demands will decrease as he learns that there is a constancy in his life. First he learns that someone comes when he calls. And second he discovers that if he waits, someone brings him good things at regular intervals—such as food, clean diapers, and secure arms to lie in.

Bringing a baby into your home will undoubtedly make big changes in your lives. No longer two individuals able to go your separate ways, you and your wife are now parents responsible for the welfare and the future of another human being. It is a big responsibility.

Husband and Wife Reports

New parents are often the most enthusiastic proselytizers of prepared childbirth. On the following pages are the postpartum reports of a couple who chose to have their child by prepared childbirth. It is worth reading them, not only for the excitement of reliving their labor with them, but also to see how each one, mother and father, perceives the progress and details of labor and delivery.

HUSBAND'S REPORT

Am dictating this letter about thirty hours after J. has delivered a baby boy, five pounds, eleven ounces at 3:19 P.M. on December 12. We went to bed rather late on Friday night, December 11, and the first time I knew J. was in labor was at about 1:15 A.M. when her bag of waters broke and she had bloody show. J. claims that the bag of waters actually broke with a kind of pop, and a few seconds later she started leaking.

The previous advice we had to lay down a rubber sheet was very good in this instance. J. went to the bathroom and stuffed a towel between her legs to try to soak up some of the liquid and blood that was coming out. J. told me at that time she thought she was having contractions about every fifteen minutes or so, and she also said she had probably been having contractions for about an hour and a half to two hours before the bag of waters actually broke.

At this point J. called our obstetrician, Dr. A., as he had directed her to do if her bag of waters broke, when she had bloody show, or when her contractions were between five to seven minutes apart. Unfortunately, Dr. A. was out, and he had given another doctor's name to his answering service. The answering service put us through to Dr. B. at about 1:30 A.M. Because J. was not really having any regular contractions at this time, Dr. B. suggested that she remain at home until her contractions became more definite. He suggested that she call him again when her contractions were about five minutes apart.

J. decided that she was going to have some trouble sleeping, and she also thought that she might toss and turn the rest of the night. Thus J. and I decided to make up the guest bed in the den, and J. decided to spend the night in the den in that bed. Another reason that she didn't stay in the same bed was that there was a bit of wetness and a mess on her side of our king size bed in the bedroom. She also wanted to be sure that I got enough sleep so that I wouldn't get cranky at any time during her labor.

At about 2:00 A.M. I went back to bed leaving J. in the den. I had some difficulty getting to sleep and I got to sleep at about 3:00 A.M. J. came in to wake me at about 4:15 A.M. and said she was a little bit concerned because she had very irregular contractions, and she thought that they were coming at about two minutes or so. I was rather sleepy at the time, but I suggested that these were probably not very severe contractions as she didn't feel any particular pain or need to do any breathing at this time. J. decided to go back to the den and wait a little longer to see what would develop. Actually, she didn't spend very much time in bed as she was making hard boiled eggs and preparing some sandwiches for me to eat at the hospital because she didn't think I would be able to get much food there if I was in the labor room with her.

I went back to sleep, and I woke up at about 6:30 A.M. when I heard J. talking on the phone with Dr. B. J. really did not know exactly how far she had progressed in labor, and Dr. B. suggested that she go on to the hospital and have them examine her and then call the doctor back.

We got to the hospital about 7:00 A.M. and we found the hospital tour that had been suggested a very good idea because we were able to park right at the emergency entrance and leave the car there and then walk into the hospital and we knew exactly where to go to the labor and delivery area. A nurse came up to greet us as we walked into the labor and delivery area, and the nurse told me to go have a seat in the waiting room while J. was being examined.

Evidently Dr. B. had called ahead to tell them that we were coming because the nurse knew our name. After waiting about an hour or perhaps a little less in the father's waiting room, a nurse came into the room and asked for me and told me that I could go into the labor room with J. I explained that I didn't know what labor room she was in because I just thought that she was going to be examined and perhaps sent home. But the nurse told me that she was going to stay at the hospital and directed me to the labor room in which J. was located. I asked J. what had been going on for the last forty-five minutes to an hour when I got into the room, and she said that she had had an enema and she had been about three-quarters shaved. She had also been examined and was apparently about two centimeters dilated.

I had brought along my stopwatch, and I tried to time J.'s contractions and also the time between contractions, but I was not able to do a very effective job because her contractions were not really very even in length or spacing. Since I was a bit hungry at this time I told J. that I would like to go down to the coffee shop and get breakfast, and she told me to go on ahead because it didn't look as if too much would be happening in the next hour.

When I came back from breakfast J. told me that Dr. B. had been in and had examined her. J. said that the examination had shown that she was three centimeters dilated. I started timing J. and her contractions were coming anywhere from one minute to about six to seven minutes apart. J. found during this time that for some contractions she didn't need to use breathing techniques at all. For some other contractions she did a funny kind of breathing exercise, which was somewhere in between a cleansing breath and breathing for the first phase of the first stage. These breaths could best be described as shallow cleansing breaths taken about every three seconds or so.

At around 11:00 A.M. her contractions seemed to be getting a little more regular. The contractions were coming at about three minute intervals. I just can't recall now whether she was continuing the shallow cleansing breaths or whether she was having to do some panting at about every third or fourth contraction. That is to say, every third or fourth contraction seemed to require a slightly higher level of breathing exercise.

Our regular obstetrician, Dr. A., came to the hospital at about 11:00 A.M. He didn't give J. a cervix examination at this time, but he stayed in the labor room for about ten minutes while J. had two or three contractions. J. described to the doctor at that time the contractions as between mild and medium rather than strong.

Over the next two hours, the contractions continued in the same vein, coming as little as one minute apart and as much as seven and a half minutes apart. From about 10:00 A.M. on, J. complained of what she thought was back labor. After the 11:00 A.M. check by Dr. A., she tried several of the suggested positions for back labor, but none of them seemed to really help much.

The best position was when the head of the bed was raised to its maximum or near its maximum point. J. would lie back between contractions and when she felt a contraction coming on, she would sit up in tailor position until the contraction was finished.

By 1:00 P.M. we were getting a little curious as to whether any progress had been made. When the nurse came in for a check at that time, we asked if we might have someone make a measurement to see if there had been any progress. The doctor came in and as before I was asked to leave the room during his examination.

I talked with the doctor outside the labor room after he completed his examination, and he said he had found that she was five centimeters dilated at this time. He also said he had found a second bag of waters in his examination and he had apparently broken the second bag of waters. I mentioned that the progress had been rather slow between three and five centimeters, but he reassured me by saying once J. was five to seven centimeters dilated the delivery would take place in a very short time thereafter.

I do recall now that shortly before 1:00 P.M., J. had become a little bit nauseous and had vomited or spit out a small amount of fluid. J. has since commented that when she tried the knee-chest position for back labor at the same time that she was doing her panting that she became somewhat nauseous.

About fifteen minutes after the doctor's examination was over, I suggested to J. that her contractions seemed to be more regular when she stayed in the position that I mentioned above, namely leaning back in between contractions and sitting up in the tailor position during contractions.

We were both getting a little bit tired and perhaps even a little bit bored at this point in time, and we were somewhat discouraged by the small amount of progress between 9:00 A.M. and 1:00 P.M. I don't know if it was the fact that the doctor had broken the bag of waters or if J. was staying in one position or what the reason was, but about 1:15 A.M. her contractions started being very regular, between two and three minutes apart, and were becoming much stronger, lasting for, in some cases, about one and a quarter minutes.

During this period J. used the panting almost exclusively during the contractions, at least during their peak. In some cases she would slow down at about forty-five seconds and use her shallow cleansing breathing, or whatever you would want to call it. In some cases she found that she still needed to do a little more panting after that, but her policy seemed to be that she would use the panting only as it was necessary and then change to this other kind of breathing as soon as she could in the contractions.

The doctor came in again at about 2:00 P.M. and found that J. was eight centimeters dilated. When I came into the room after the examination, I told J. that this was going to be the difficult period and that I hoped that we could get through it all right. Outside in the hall the doctor had told me that J. was only about forty-five minutes away from being able to start pushing and I told J. this in the hope that it would encourage her. In the next forty-five minutes the contractions were running about every two minutes and in some cases about a minute to a minute and a half apart.

The contractions seemed to be almost classic transition contractions in that they would peak almost immediately (within the first five seconds) and continue somewhat erratically over the next minute to minute and a half. J. panted quite vigorously during this transition period, and her panting increased every time the contraction seemed to be peaking. The nurse came in at about 2:30 P.M. and we told her the contractions were becoming quite strong. She said to be sure to call her and that she would get the doctor as soon as J. felt the urge to push. After about three more strong contractions J. pushed the buzzer to call the nurse because she thought she did feel the urge to push at that time.

The doctor's examination showed that J. was about ten centimeters dilated and that she could start pushing at any time. J. gave a couple of pushes while the doctor was in there and then I came into the labor room. At this point the sheet had been taken off her legs so that I could watch for the baby's head. The nurse told me to call her if I could see the baby's head. After about three contractions I did see the head or what I thought was the baby's head, and I called the nurse. She came into the room and watched J. push for one contraction, and then she called the doctor in and he said she was just about ready to go into the delivery room. J. was wheeled into the delivery room at around 3:00 P.M.

The doctor took me to a room and had me change into a surgical gown or some kind of sterilized or sanitized gown so that I could be in the delivery room. I also at this time had to sign a form which allowed me to go into the delivery room. The doctor told me to wait by the nurses' station until I was called into the delivery room. I waited what seemed an eternity but probably was only about two or three minutes. I was afraid that J. was going to have the baby before I could get into the delivery room and I asked the nurse on the station how I would be called into the delivery room. She said that a nurse would come out and get me. About one minute later the nurse did come out, and I went into the delivery room. A stool had been set up for me right next to J.'s head.

There was a convenient mirror on the wall so that J. could see the baby being born and by putting my head close to J.'s I could also see in this mirror. J. had asked me to bring her glasses into the room with me. I did that and she put them on. Otherwise she would have been unable to see in the mirror. Shortly after I got into the delivery room the doctor gave J. a local anesthetic because he was about to perform an episiotomy.

As J. had a contraction, the doctor performed the episiotomy.

J. did a good job pushing and I encouraged her. After the doctor completed the episiotomy, we waited until the next contraction and the doctor and I encouraged J. to give a good hard push. She did and then fell back to get strength and breath for the next push. The doctor told her to push, but she said the urge had gone away. About two seconds later she said that she had the urge again, and we both encouraged her to push. The baby's head was born on that push.

The doctor immediately took the head in his hands and cleaned out the mouth. I can't recall now, but I don't think that J. ever really gave another good strong push for the rest of the baby's delivery but I could be mistaken in this. She will probably remember better. It just seems that it wasn't very long after the baby's head was born that the doctor lifted out the whole baby and exclaimed, "It's a boy!" I said to J. at about that time, "Well there is Norris, our new son!" The baby weighed in at five pounds, eleven ounces and was nineteen inches in length and even had a little bit of red hair along with the blood.

After the baby was born, I told J. that the most difficult part was coming up because the doctor had to sew up the episiotomy. But because he had used the anesthetic for the incision, it turned out that J. really didn't feel the stitches at all. The placenta came out within five minutes, perhaps even less, after the baby was born. After the doctor had finished the stitching and had cleaned up J. a little bit, he showed us the placenta in detail.

A book that J. and I had read just the night before Norris was born had helped me understand a little bit more about what would go on in the delivery room. The name of the book is *The Birth of a Child*. It is published by Crown Publishers, Inc. in New York and is primarily a set of photographs of a delivery. The text is by Ann Dally. I recommend this book strongly for people taking the classes.

Both J. and I were very happy using the Lamaze method, and I must say that I did make a comment in the delivery room that it was rather amazing. I think I said, "It's unbelievable" because it was difficult for me to believe that the child I had just seen born was mine and J's. After the delivery of the placenta J. was given a shot to help her uterus to contract. At that point I went out of the delivery room and changed into my street clothes while J. was being wheeled to her room. The baby was turned over to the nurses there.

Well, it's now been about thirty hours or so, thirty-two hours perhaps, since Norris was born, and J. seems to be in very fine condition. J. is able to walk around, is not dopey in any way. She has had some pills to help her uterus contract, and she also has taken some codeine-based pain killers because she has had some cramps in her uterus. But all in all I think she is in very good condition.

We are both extremely happy with the Lamaze method, and J. has said to me that she didn't think she could have made it without my assistance. She said the contractions that she had during transition when Dr. A. was in the room and I was not there were much more difficult than the contractions that she had when I was present and counting off the seconds with the stopwatch.

Sincerely,
B.

WIFE'S REPORT

We are writing to thank you for your help in preparing us for labor and delivery and to tell you about our very happy outcome. We have a new son, Norris, born at 3:19 P.M. Saturday, December 12. He was a bit small, weighing five pounds, eleven ounces, nineteen inches long, and his pediatrician says he is healthy and well. We hope he will continue to be so.

B. has recorded his comments and impressions and his version of the labor. Since I've not yet seen his record, mine will in large part duplicate his, I'm afraid, but it will be a different point of view.

I last saw my doctor at a regular visit on Monday, December 7. He said my cervix was a bit effaced, but not very much and that the baby really hadn't begun to engage yet. Thus he said he wouldn't be at all surprised to see me in his office for another visit the next Monday.

On Tuesday my Braxton-Hicks contractions started to become much more frequent and intense. Some of them even began to be painful slightly, in the groin area. So I suspected that I might well not make it to Monday next after all. Thursday night they were quite frequent and I even began to think labor might be starting, but then they faded and went away.

About 11:00 P.M. on Friday, December 11, the supposed due date, I started to have contractions that seemed as if they might be the real thing, although I was confused because they felt like a tightening of the groin and bladder area rather than a pulling together of the uterine muscle as the early Braxton-Hicks had. Indeed, this was one aspect of labor which really did surprise me—the way in which I felt the contractions. Once labor was underway, I never really was aware of tightening of the uterus, except as I felt it with my hand—i.e., externally.

Since I wasn't sure, and the intervals were fifteen to twenty minutes, I didn't say anything to B. and we went to bed normally. Indeed, we even practiced breathing as usual, fortunately for me, concentrating on the panting which had been giving me some trouble in the last few weeks. We *thought* we had it straightened out and as it turned out we did.

About twenty minutes after lights out, 12:45 to 1:00 A.M. I felt a distinct contraction which suddenly ended with a "pop." I don't know if I actually heard it or only felt it, but it was very definite. I wondered for about two seconds if that were the membranes, and then there was no question. Fortunately we had a rubber sheet on the bed as you suggested and I had a towel at my head. I grabbed it up and stuffed it between my legs and took off for the bathroom. There was a good quantity of fluid and some bloody show but not a great deal. B. of course was awake again at this point. I called my doctor, as he had told me to, and he was off for the weekend! I was turned over to the fellow he had taking his calls for him. He said to try to go back to bed and wait until I was sure true labor was underway, and then call him back.

Since my side of the bed was a mess and since I wanted B. to get as much sleep as he could so as to be wide awake later when he would be needed, we made up the spare bed for me in the study, and I moved in there with a supply of towels to catch my leaking.

One suggestion I would make—have a *good* supply of old towels or something to catch the leak on hand. I was nervous about making a mess of the mattress and so did not relax as well as I might have, thus missing some sleep I might have gotten.

The contractions pretty well stopped for about the next hour and then started coming very raggedly about every two or three minutes. I used a stopwatch to time—much better than a sweep second hand because you don't have to watch it—just punch the stop. These early contractions were very confusing and irregular, though extremely mild. They lasted as long as 90-100 seconds and were quite close together. I found that I felt them most intensely while on my side, and almost not at all while standing. Certainly no breathing was needed to control them.

After about an hour of sitting or lying in bed—flat was also a good position—I decided that since obviously this was real I'd best get prepared. I got up and made B. some sandwiches and hard boiled some eggs for his breakfast. Then I read for a while.

About 4:00 A.M. I started to be concerned because the contractions, despite being very mild, were so close together and long lasting. So I went in and woke B., and asked his advice. He said use my judgment and call the doctor when it seemed best. So I left him in bed and decided to wait a bit more myself. They certainly weren't hurting so long as I didn't lie on my side although I was *beginning* to feel something in my back.

In bed I tried to doze a bit and finally about 6:30 A.M. called the doctor again. He reassured me that labor sometimes did start with very long, closely spaced, mild cramps and suggested I come to the hospital to be checked for progress. He said I could go home again if the progress were too little (we live about one mile from the hospital).

So I woke B. again and told him we were off. My suitcase was all ready, as was my brown paper bag, so we simply had to get dressed. As I stupidly had no Kotex, I had to use a pad of Kleenex to catch the leak.

Our hospital tour a month earlier had shown us just where to go so there was no confusion when we arrived. The doctor had called ahead, so the nurse was expecting us. I was checked in at 7:10 A.M. and told that I would have to stay since my membranes had ruptured. B. had been sent off to the waiting room while I was prepared. The nurse shaved me, but only partially fortunately and then the usual enema. Since my contractions were still very mild, it was no real problem and not really nearly as unpleasant as I had anticipated. She then examined me and said I was two centimeters dilated.

When this was done, the nurses left me alone. Finally I rang the bell and asked them to get B., which was done. He had been waiting all this time not even knowing I was to stay. That was the *only* problem we had with the hospital the whole time there. I told the nurses I was prepared, and they just left us alone.

When B. came in, my contractions were still very mild and now seemed more widely spaced. I still didn't need any breathing techniques. So B. went off and got a newspaper and then had breakfast. He was gone about an hour, during which I read the paper and ignored the contractions which were becoming a bit stronger.

About 9:00 A.M. the doctor who was subbing for my doctor came in and examined me. I thought he said I was four centimeters dilated (later I learned I was three centimeters at this point, a trivial difference but pschologically valuable since I was encouraged then about progress, and *later,* four hours later when it was only five centimeters, I then had gone from three to five).

All this time I continued to leak and have bloody show but was very relaxed about it because I figured the hospital was set to cope with it. In this sense I was much more relaxed at the hospital than at home.

About 9:30 A.M. I began to feel a need to use the first phase breathing. Very shortly that was not enough and I switched to panting, but found an improvisation that helped preserve strength. Rather than panting all the way through a contraction, I would start panting and then as it eased off, switch to a fast, shallow breathing. At this point the contractions lasted about sixty seconds and were at irregular intervals of two to four minutes. They also varied in intensity, and it was frequently hard to be sure when one had ended. About half felt in lower groin, about half in lower back.

About 10:30 A.M. my regular doctor came in. He had been called by the other doctor before he got off on a hunting trip, and he took over from then on. He stayed for about ten minutes to feel some contractions with me but I didn't have any good ones while he was there (naturally!). So he left for a while.

Increasingly the contractions were in the back and I stopped all effleurage and put my fists in the back. A semi-sitting position seemed to be the best. About 11:00 A.M. a nurse came in and offered some medication which I refused—no need.

Although you had said and we had read that there was complete relief between contractions, I did not find this to be the case. Through the morning the contractions were more and more in the back, and I continued to feel some tension sensation there between them. This made it particularly hard to know when a contraction had stopped.

Several times I tried the back labor positions, but none of them seemed as good as the semi-sitting position with the hospital bed rolled almost all the way up.

Since no one had said anything to the contrary, I got out of bed several times; tried standing and moving about a bit. It seemed to relieve my tension (and I was more tense than I would have wished) but B. seemed to feel that it slowed the contractions down. I'm not sure he was right.

About 1:00 P.M. I rang the buzzer and asked to be examined since I'd had no progress report since 9:00 A.M. My doctor came in and surprisingly found a protrusion like a bag of water. He ruptured it. It turned out I had had two membranes (made the placenta look strange as we later found), but at this point I was only five centimeters dilated. That seemed a bit discouraging, but the doctor told B. he thought I would progress fast now.

He was right. The contractions became increasingly strong and never really seemed to stop. One hundred percent in the back at this point. The panting continued to control. I never felt that I might lose control of a specific contraction although at times I wasn't sure how many more I would be able to handle.

By now I was actually *dozing* between contractions, then coming awake with a cleansing breath. B. too was dozing and would punch the pin on his stopwatch with my breath. It was practically impossible to tell when a contraction stopped; they just deteriorated to a lower back ache.

At 2:00 P.M. the doctor came in again, checked and said I was eight centimeters dilated. He said I'd probably be ready to push in less than an hour and offered me a drug of some sort to relax. I told him I'd been dozing between contractions and thought I could handle it. He said fine, it was up to me. And to buzz the nurses when I thought I felt an urge to push.

I should note that the hardest time I had controlling contractions was when the doctor was examining me, flat on my back. In particular, I didn't have B. there to count off the seconds and I really missed that. Occasionally I was feeling slightly sick while panting, but nothing came of it so long as I had a bedpan nearby —psychological I guess, because I found it very disturbing not to have it available. The doctor said it was probably because I was hyperventilating.

After the doctor left, the contractions really started to be strong. I tried switching to transition breathing, but it did not seem to work as well as straight panting, so I resumed that. I never did use the transition breathing after that.

By now I'd stopped dozing between contractions and was really concentrating on them. They got very strong, seemed to peak at about five and fifteen seconds. B. was giving me a five second count and that helped. Lasted anywhere up to two minutes. After several very strong contractions, which I almost felt lift me up off the bed, I thought maybe I was feeling an urge to push or if I weren't, I should be. It never was definite and sure. So I buzzed the doctor and he came in; said the cervix was all gone and I could push.

This was sometime between 2:30 and 2:45 P.M. They sent B. out to get changed and again I was all alone. The bed had been left flat so I got a nurse to come in and raise it. She started to tell me how to push, then saw that I knew how so said to go my own way. B. came back and the nurse said to call her when B. could see some head.

Once I started pushing all the back pain seemed to disappear, at least it seemed that way. It wasn't comfortable, nor easy, but it was doing something on which I could concentrate hard. After about two or three contractions B. thought he saw head so he called the doctor and nurse. They came in and sent him off to finish getting changed. Then I had to sign a release form for having B. in the delivery room—hardly the ideal time, and my signature was a bit shaky to say the least.

The labor room bed was wheeled into the delivery room, no transfer problem there. In the delivery room the doctor had them put a triangular wedge on the table for a back prop. It worked very well. There were no stirrups and I asked for them and they were put on. I suspect they do use them most of the time. The table also had bars for me to grasp with my hands (I was warned to keep them under the drape). The transfer from the labor room bed to the delivery table got fouled and I wound up on my hands and knees facing the head of the table. Somehow we got me flopped over between contractions and I continued to push as they came. The mirror was adjusted so I could see and then, finally, B. came in.

About two contractions and an episiotomy later, we had the baby, at 3:19 P.M. The placenta detached almost at once and another push had it out. The doctor sewed up the incision at once (after getting the baby going—he cried almost at once, on his own) so the same local he had given me for the cut served for the stitches. No real pain with them.

After the baby was cleaned up, the nurse gave him to me to hold and the doctor showed us the placenta. I was feeling really great now and was making various dubious jokes.

Total time in the delivery room, from in the door to out, was twenty-nine minutes. They had me in my room and all cleaned up in no time, and B. and I called my parents before 4:00 P.M. They were a bit surprised by the quickness, to say the least.

By 5:30 P.M. I'd had dinner and still couldn't go to sleep. Didn't really make it until late that night.

All in all we were delighted with how things went and want to thank you very much for your help.

Sincerely,

J.

Labor Review Charts

PRELIMINARY PHASE

Duration: zero to many hours.

Contractions are: mild; lasting thirty to forty seconds, from five to twenty minutes apart; usually felt from the back, radiating frontwards.

Work being done by these contractions: early effacement.

Mood: happy, excited, "labor is finally here."

Other symptoms: show; if membranes are ruptured, there may be a steady trickle of clear, odorless fluid; awareness of backache.

Techniques

Conserve energy; if possible, sleep; if not, keep busy but do not overtire; drink sweet, clear fluids as allowed; try different positions for comfort.

Husband's role

Get as much rest as possible. Assist wife to find comfortable position. Remind her to empty bladder. Begin labor record.

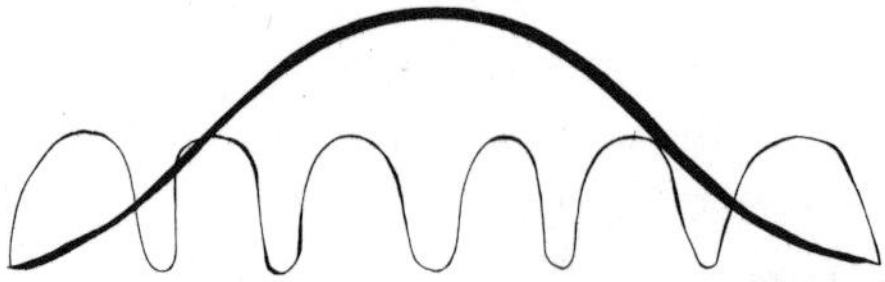

Diagram 1. *EARLY ACTIVE PHASE: This contraction in labor will last for thirty to forty seconds. Breathing should be slow and rhythmic at a rate of about eight breaths per minute plus deep breaths at beginning and end of contraction. Do not begin until needed.*

EARLY ACTIVE PHASE

Duration: two to six hours.

Contractions are: moderate; lasting thirty to forty seconds, from five to ten minutes apart.

Work being done by these contractions: completion of effacement; dilation from one to four centimeters.

Mood: confident this is true labor; still talkative.

Other symptoms: nothing new.

Techniques

Conserve energy; controlled relaxation; slow rhythmic chest breathing when necessary; accelerate only as needed; use comfort positions.

Husband's role

Call doctor; time contractions; check wife for tension; encourage her to empty bladder; rest as much as possible; eat even though wife cannot by now.

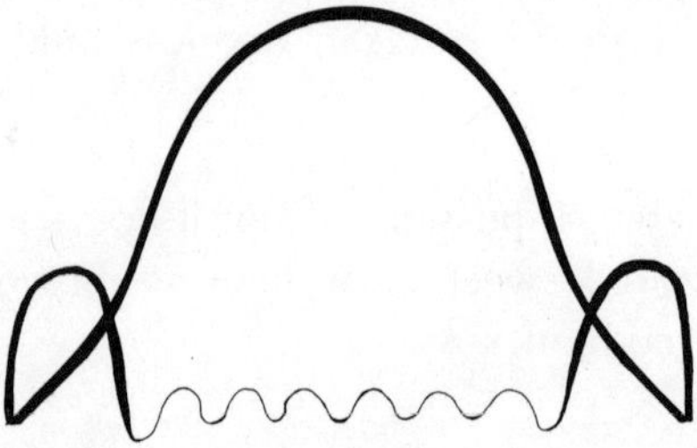

Diagram 2. *ACTIVE PHASE: Shallow breathing should be used as necessary when slow rhythmic chest breathing is no longer effective.*

ACTIVE PHASE

Duration: two to three hours.

Contractions are: strong; lasting fifty to sixty seconds, from three to five minutes apart, each reaching a definite peak.

Work being done by these contractions: dilation of cervix from five to eight centimeters.

Other symptoms: sudden gush if membranes rupture, leading to intensification of contractions.

Techniques

Conserve energy; controlled relaxation. When chest breathing is no longer effective, progress to accelerated-decelerated shallow breathing. Make changes only as necessary. Determine techniques by the way contractions feel, not by the place in labor.

Husband's role

Take wife to hospital during this phase. "Count down" contractions; remind wife to empty bladder; offer mouth rinses and cool cloth for face. Use tactile cues—touch, stroke arms, legs; rub back. Talk to wife; keep her informed. Keep personnel informed. Keep labor record.

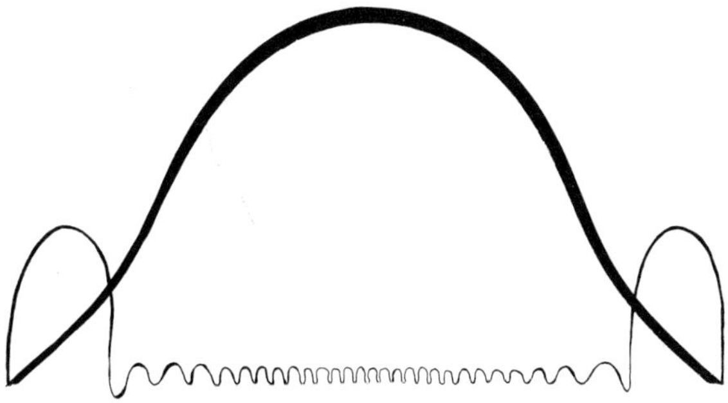

Diagram 3. *ACTIVE PHASE: When shallow breathing is no longer enough, switch to accelerated-decelerated shallow breathing and effleurage.*

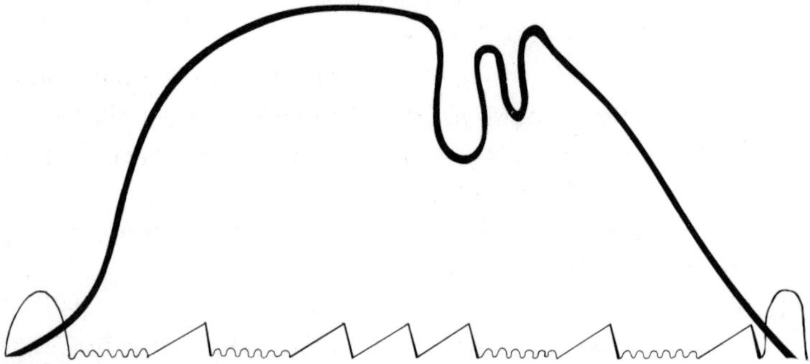

Diagram 4. *TRANSITION: The breathing for transition must be rhythmic. You can vary the rhythm from six pants and a blow to four pants and a blow—whatever provides your wife with the most control during this short, difficult phase. All blows should be short, staccato.*

TRANSITION

Duration: twenty to forty-five minutes.

Contractions are: strong; erratic; may have peaks lasting sixty to ninety seconds, from thirty seconds to two minutes apart.

Work being done by these contractions: final dilation of cervix from eight to ten centimeters.

Mood: irritable; ready to give up.

Other symptoms: difficulty relaxing; inability to communicate; chills; trembling of muscles; nausea; vomiting; backache; rectal pressure.

Techniques

Pant-blow breathing during contractions; slow rhythmic breathing in between; work at relaxation.

Husband's role

Encourage wife; take one contraction at a time; remind her baby is almost here. Give precise directions. When she has the urge to push, tell her to "Blow . . . blow . . . blow." Get doctor between contractions.

DELIVERY, OR EXPULSION

Duration: ten to sixty minutes.

Contractions are: strong, rhythmic; lasting sixty to ninety seconds, from three to five minutes apart.

Work being done by these contractions: pushing the baby from inside to outside.

Mood: refreshed; energetic.

Techniques

Push effectively with contraction; relax and slow breathe in between. Stop pushing on doctor's command to ease delivery of head.

Husband's role

Assist wife with position for expulsion, check technique and verbal cues while still in labor room. In delivery room, cue for technique and relay doctor's orders. Keep wife informed of progress.

Suggested Readings

Castor, Constance. *Participating in Childbirth: A Parents' Guide.* Farmingdale, New York: Privately Published, 1971.

An excellent supplement to classes in prepared childbirth. Offers a concise review of all class material and a guide to the labor process for fathers. Available through ASPO, 7 West 96th Street, New York City 10025.

Chabon, Irwin. *Awake and Aware: Participation in Childbirth through Psychoprophylaxis.* New York: Dell Publishing Co., 1969.

A good book on the theory behind the psychoprophylaxis method. Explains complex scientific ideas in easily understood terms. Available in paperback.

Flanagan, Geraldine L. *The First Nine Months of Life.* New York: Simon and Schuster, 1962.

A fascinating, pictorial study of life before birth. Available in paperback.

Maternity Center Association. *A Baby Is Born*. New York: Grosset and Dunlap, Inc., 1964.

A text and pictorial presentation of the processes of conception through delivery. A good resource book that relies on the medical sculptures of Dickinson and Belskie to illustrate the text. Available from Maternity Center Association, 48 East 92nd Street, New York City 10028.

Maury, Marian, ed. *Birth Right and Birth Rate*. New York: MacFadden Books, 1963.

A philosophical look at responsible parenthood. Available in paperback.

Salk, Lee and Kramer, Rita. *How to Raise a Human Being: A Parents' Guide to Emotional Health from Infancy through Adolescence*. New York: Random House, 1969.

An excellent guide for parents.

Stender, Fay, ed. *Husbands in the Delivery Room*. Bellevue, Wash.: International Childbirth Education Association, 1965.

A good source of information and statistics for allowing husbands to be in the delivery room. Available from ICEA, 208 Ditty Building, Bellevue, Washington 98004.

Velley, Pierre. *Childbirth with Confidence*. Translated by Elliot E. Philip. New York: Macmillian Co., 1969.

This book recognizes that the husband does have an important role to play in childbearing, not perhaps as active as in this country but a role nevertheless.

Glossary

abdominal: pertaining to the abdomen.

afterbirth: the third stage of labor and delivery in which all the structures necessary during pregnancy but no longer necessary after the birth of the baby are expelled by the body—the remainder of the membranes, the placenta, and the cord which is still attached to it. Also, **secundines.**

amenorrhea: the absence of menstrual discharge.

amnesia: loss of memory.

amnion: membrane which contains the waters surrounding the baby in utero. Also, **amniotic sac.**

analgesia: relief from pain without loss of consciousness.

androgen: any substance which produces masculine characteristics, such as the testicular hormone.

anesthesia: loss of sensation.

anoxia: oxygen deficiency; of particular concern when referring to the unborn baby, i.e., **fetal anoxia.**

antenatal: anything which occurs before birth. Also, **ante partum, prenatal.**

areola: pigmented area surrounding the nipple of the breast.

attitude: the position of the fetus in the uterus.

bag of waters: amniotic sac.

Braxton-Hicks contractions: painless uterine contractions, occurring throughout pregnancy, early to accommodate the growing fetus, later to prepare the cervix for labor to begin. Also, **false labor.**

breech delivery: delivery of fetus with buttocks or feet first.
caput succedaneum: a swelling that may appear on the presenting part of the fetus. It is caused by pressure during labor and delivery and will disappear by itself.
caudal: a form of spinal anesthesia introduced into the caudal canal, considered to be below the actual spinal cord.
cephalic: relating to the head.
cervix: the necklike part of the uterus which must become thin and open before the baby can be born.
Caesarian section: delivery of the baby through the abdominal and uterine walls by surgery.
circumcision: the removal of all or part of the prepuce, or foreskin, of the penis. May be done by a pediatrician or in a ritual ceremony if the family is of the Jewish faith.
coitus: sexual intercourse. Also, **copulation.**
colostrum: the substance that precedes the production of milk in the mother's breast. Colostrum is said to be valuable to the baby as a source of easily digested protein and as a laxative. Colostrum is also thought to transmit immunizing agents from mother to baby.
conception: the union of a spermatozoon and an ovum to produce, eventually, another being.
confinement: old term used to describe the labor and delivery period.
congenital: present at birth.
dystocia: difficult, slow, or painful delivery; usually requires obstetrical intervention.
effacement: the thinning and shortening of the cervix during labor.
engagement: entrance of the fetus into the beginning of the birth canal; the largest diameter of the presenting part fits itself into the largest diameter of the pelvis. Once there, it usually does not disengage.
engorgement: the condition which occurs in conjunction with lactation in which the breasts become temporarily hard and tender. This condition will clear itself as lactation continues.
episiotomy: a surgical incision of the perineum for the purpose of enlarging the external opening.
erythroblastosis fetalis: a severe hemolytic disease of the newborn usually due to blood incompatibility. Also, **Rh-disease.**
estrogen: a substance which produces female characteristics; it is secreted by the ovaries and placenta.
Fallopian tubes: the oviducts, or tubes from the uterus which open near the ovaries and receive the ovum.

fetus: the baby from the end of the fifth week of pregnancy until birth.

fontanel: the diamond-shaped space between the frontal and parietal bones in the infant, just above the forehead. There is also a fontanel between the occiput and parietal bones, at the back of the baby's head. Also, **soft spot.**

fundus: the upper, rounded part of the uterus.

gravida: a pregnant woman.

hormone: a chemical substance secreted by one organ in the body which causes other organs to act.

in utero: inside the uterus.

involution: the process by which the uterus returns to its normal size and position after birth, usually requiring about six weeks.

labor: the process by which the cervix effaces and dilates from zero to ten centimeters.

lactation: 1. the time during which a mother is secreting milk; 2. the process of secretion of milk.

lanugo: fine, downy hair covering found on nearly all parts of fetus except palms of the hands and soles of the feet.

lochia: vaginal discharge following birth, starting out red and progressing to a brown color then to a white.

milia: the white dots often seen across the nose of the newborn, caused by blocked sebaceous glands.

molding: the shaping of the baby's head so that it can fit through the birth passages.

multipara: a woman who has had several children.

navel: the umbilicus; belly button.

neonatal: newborn.

ovary: female sex organ which produces eggs.

ovulation: the discharge of an ovum from the ovary.

ovum: a single female reproductive cell. Also, **egg.**

oxytocin: hormone secreted by the pituitary gland which stimulates uterine contractions.

parity: a woman's past history regarding childbearing.

parturient: the woman in childbirth.

parturition: the process of childbirth.

perineum: the area between the vagina and the rectum.

placenta: the organ which supports the life functions of the fetus.

pre-eclampsia: a dangerous complication of pregnancy which can threaten the lives of both mother and baby. Symptoms are high blood pressure, excessive weight gain, edema, headaches.

premature infant: any infant weighing less than 2500 grams at birth.

presentation: the position of the fetus as determined by the part of his body that is felt at the time of internal examination, i.e., **vertex, breech.**

primipara: a woman who has given birth to her first child.

puerperium: the approximate six-week period from delivery to the the return of the uterus to its normal position.

secundines: the afterbirth.

show: the blood-tinged mucus discharged from the vagina usually signalling the beginning of labor.

umbilicus: the cord or lifeline which connects the fetus with the placenta, provides the fetus with nutrients and oxygen, and removes wastes to the maternal system for elimination.

vernix caseosa: "cheesy" substance that protects the skin of the fetus in utero.

vertex presentation: fetal presentation where the top of the head is the presenting part.

zygote: the cell produced when the ovum and spermatozoon unite.

Index